The Ocular Fundus

Methods of Examination and Typical Findings

Professor **ARNO NOVER**, M.D.

Director of the University Eye Clinic in Mainz

Translated from the German by FREDERICK C. BLODI, M.D.
Professor and Head, Department of Ophthalmology,
The University of Iowa, College of Medicine, Iowa City, Iowa.

Third, new and enlarged edition

With 112 color and 42 black and white illustrations

LEA & FEBIGER 1974 PHILADELPHIA

Preface to Third Edition

The text was improved and complemented for the third edition. The chapter on "Diseases of the Vitreous" has been added.

Numerous improvements are based on letters by critical readers. I would like to express my special thanks to all of them.

The publishing company has shown a most understanding cooperation once again. They have responded to all of my wishes and I would thank them cordially.

Mainz, April 1974   A. NOVER

Preface to First Edition

This book should be a supplement to lectures and courses in ophthalmology for the medical student, for the practicing physician it should be a helping guide for treating his patients. We hope it will make it easier for them to learn the techniques of examination and to evaluate the ophthalmoscopic findings.

For this reason we have put into the center of our discussion the description of the most important and practical methods of examination, and the illustration of the most characteristic changes of the ocular fundus.

In addition to findings which are predominantly of ophthalmologic interest we have discussed those in which the fundus changes are part of a systemic disease.

The next is short and discusses only those points which are necessary for the understanding of the changes in the ocular fundus and their differential diagnosis. More detailed discussions would not fit into the framework of such a book.

I would like to express my special gratitude to my teacher, Professor K. VOM HOFF, the director of the University Eye Clinic in Cologne. His kind interest and valuable suggestions have considerably helped my work.

I would like also to thank Dozent Dr. H. TOHMANN, Oberarzt of the University Eye Clinic in Cologne for critically surveying the text, and Miss S. MAASS for her help in producing the photographs and illustrations.

I would also like to thank Mr. F. K. SCHATTAUER, the owner of the F. K. Schattauer Publishing House, who has magnanimously granted all my wishes, and has therefore, considerably contributed to the realization of my work, and has given the book an excellent format.

Cologne, Germany, March 1964   A. NOVER

Contents

GENERAL PART

I. Introduction

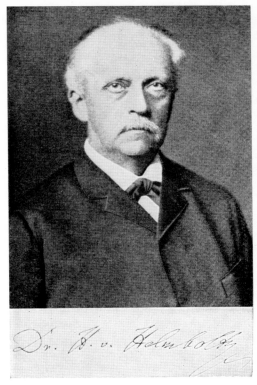

Fig. 1. H. v. HELMHOLTZ (1821–1894).

1. The Invention of the Ophthalmoscope

An examination of the ocular fundus has only been possible since the invention of the ophthalmoscope by HERRMANN VON HELMHOLTZ (Fig. 1) on December 17, 1850.

The term "ophthalmoscope" ("ocular mirror") has been used since the end of the fifteenth century for spectacles. It was also known for a long time that the eyes of various animals (cat, dog, goat, wolf, others) will light up under certain optical conditions. These eyes have, as we now know, between retina and choroid a crystal-containing cellular layer – the choroidal tapetum lucidum – which reflects light falling into the eyes. In 1735 the reflection of light from albinotic eyes was observed, but only in 1810 was it recognized that this visualization of the human ocular fundus is due to the reflection of light and is absent in darkness.

3

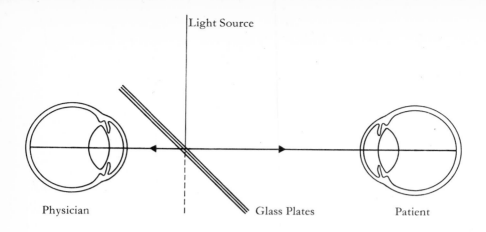

Fig. 2. Course of light rays in the original Helmholtz ophthalmoscope.

It took, however, a certain time before a useful ophthalmoscope was developed. During the 19th century especially, E. W. VON BRÜCKE, J. E. PURKINJE and H. KUSSMAUL worked on this problem. Only Helmholtz, however, recognized the fact that light falling into the eye will be reflected into the same pathway and will, therefore, reach its origin, namely the light source (conjugated points). In order to bring this reflected light into the eye of the observer his head has to be brought into the pathway of the light without obscuring the rays of the incident light. HELMHOLTZ succeeded in 1850 by using three plane-parallel, reflecting, glass plates which he brought under an angle into the common visual axis of observer and patient. In this way he could introduce himself into the pathway of the light and put himself indirectly at the light source (Fig. 2). In this way the principle of ophthalmoscopy was detected and this is still the basis of modern ophthalmoscopes (Figs. 10, 11, 13) which have undergone numerous technical improvements. Before that time all diseases of the interior of the eye were lumped together and could not be differentiated. From then on details of the interior of the eye, of the vitreous, retina and choroid, optic nervehead and the blood vessels were visible.

This new examination method became rapidly popular. ALBRECHT VON GRAEFE, one of the founders of modern ophthalmology, said that, "it opened a new world." It helped not only in the foundation and extension of ophthalmology, but it is today still the most important connection between ophthalmology and other medical specialities.

2. The Importance of Ophthalmoscopic Examination

The possibility to observe in a rather simple fashion with adequate magnification arterioles, venules and capillaries (that is the terminal part of a vascular bed) is of great importance not only for the ophthalmologist, but also for the general practitioner, the internist, the neurologist, the neurosurgeon, the pediatrician and the gynecologist. The status of the vessels allows certain conclusions as to the status of blood vessels in other organs and systems. The same is true as far as the ophthalmoscopic evaluation of the optic nerve is concerned. This nerve is nothing but an extension of brain tissue. Pathologic changes of the optic nerve may allow us to make important diagnostic conclusions as to diseases of the central nervous system.

In the following pages we discuss and illustrate not only findings of interest to the *ophthalmologist*, but also many others which are *signs of systemic diseases* and are, therefore, of importance to any physician. It has, however, to be emphasized that in every case the ophthalmoscopic finding has to be complemented by a careful history and by an evaluation of other signs and symptoms.

The examination of the eyegrounds requires practicing a special technique. The evaluation of the findings needs a certain amount of experience. A course in ophthalmoscopy should be in the curriculum of every medical school. Most practitioners lack, however, this experience and practice so that they might have difficulties in evaluating the eyeground especially when the conditions are not ideal. This may be the case in patients who are unconscious, in patients with seizures, in patients with questionable brain tumor, injuries to the skull, or sudden blindness.

For this reason we shall first describe the most important methods of ophthalmoscopy so that even the less experienced physician may be able to use this technique when examining and treating his patients.

II. Methods of Examination

The objective examination of the patient begins with the *inspection* of the eye. It is important to compare *both* eyes. For the evaluation of the anterior segment of the eye the *lateral illumination* and the *transillumination with the ophthalmoscope* are of importance. The same methods can be used to examine the refractive media, whereas ophthalmoscopy is used to view the ocular fundus.

1. Lateral Illumination

The *lateral illumination* allows a more detailed examination of the *anterior segment* of the eye (especially opacities in cornea, aqueous and lens) than the ordinary inspection in the usual, diffuse light.

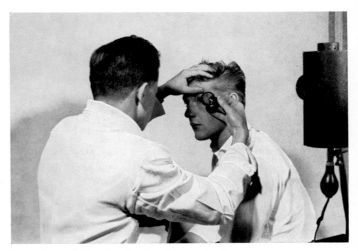

Fig. 3. Lateral illumination for the examination of the anterior segment of the eye.

The *examination* can be done in any office although a dark room may be of some advantage. The light source is held in one hand close to the head of the patient and the beam of the light is focused on the eye (Fig. 3). In this way the part of the eye to be examined will appear brightly illuminated. It is occasionally of great advantage to perform this examination while using a magnifying lens. Most convenient and advantageous is a binocular loupe which is worn like a spectacle lens. The magnification of such a loupe is between 2 × and 3 × (Figs. 4 and 5).

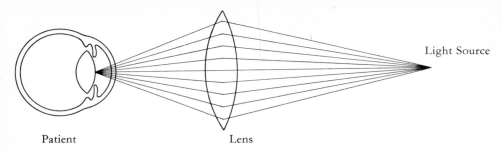

Patient   Lens   Light Source

Fig. 4. Course of light rays in focal, lateral illumination.

The principle of focal, lateral illumination is also used in the so-called slit-lamp. A strong, slit-like light source is used for lateral illumination and at the same time the anterior segment of the eye is examined with the corneal binocular microscope. With the help of additional filters or lenses the slit-lamp can also be used to examine the depth of the anterior chamber, the structure of the chamber angle (gonioscopy), the vitreous and the ocular fundus. Some ophthalmoscopes have an attachment for slit illumination.

2. Transillumination with the Ophthalmoscope

Transillumination is an examination evaluating the amount of light transmitted to the fundus. Originally a plane or concave mirror was used which had a central hole (CHR. TH. RUETE, 1851/1852). The light source had to be situated behind and somewhat to the side of the patient. At present, the direct ophthalmoscope is used for this type of examination. The ophthalmoscope is put in front of the examiner's dominant eye and the physician's head is about 3 feet away from the patient's head. It is of advantage to darken the room slightly. When the light of the ophthalmoscope is turned on, it should be directed toward the patient's pupil. No lens should be in the ophthalmoscope's disc (Fig. 5). Normally the pupil should appear diffusely red. If this is not the case, an opacity of one kind or another prevents the light from reaching the ocular fundus. Occasionally the shape of such an opacity can be evaluated by transillumination.

A more exact examination of the deeper parts of the eye evaluating lens, vitreous and the periphery of the fundus, necessitates a *dilatation of the pupil*. This is especially necessary when there are opacifications of the refractive media.

For the **dilatation of the pupil** we use **eye drops** which either stimulate the dilator muscle of the pupil (sympathicomimetic drugs) or drugs which paralyze the sphincter muscle of the pupil (parasympathicolytic drugs.)

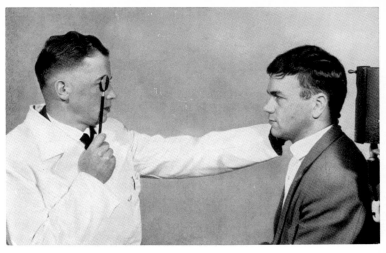

Fig. 5. Illumination with the ophthalmoscope.

For the *diagnostic* dilatation (mydriasis) we use drugs which are short-lasting and influence the accommodation as little as possible. One of the most popular drugs nowadays is Mydriacyl.

For an *objective refraction, accommodation* has to be excluded by paralyzing the ciliary muscle (cycloplegia). One of the most popular drugs for this purpose is Cyclogyl. In children Atropine may have to be used. For the therapeutic dilatation (for instance, in inflammations of the cornea or the iris or after a cataract extraction) Scopolamine or Atropine are the drugs of choice.

Occasionally, we have to forgo mydriasis, as for instance if the patient has a tendency for angle closure glaucoma or when there is a suspicion of an intracranial hemorrhage. In the first condition, dilatation of the pupil could block the chamber angle and produce a dangerous increase in the intraocular pressure (angle closure glaucoma). In the latter conditions, the observation of the pupils and their reactions is an indication to the general condition of the patient. The increase of intracranial pressure may manifest itself in the pupil and the indication for a surgical intervention may depend upon this examination.

a) Localization of Opacities of the Refractive Media

The lateral illumination is sufficient to localize accurately an opacification of the *anterior* segment (page 10). If the opacification lies *deeper*, for instance in the *lens* or the *vitreous*, we have to use the ophthalmoscope for transillumination and the parallactic shift produced by moving the eye (Fig. 6). If we, for instance, ask the patient to look down, opacities lying in the *pupillary plane* (anterior lens surface) (2) will not change their position. On the other hand, opacities lying *behind the pupillary plane*, for instance near the posterior surface of the lens (3) or in the

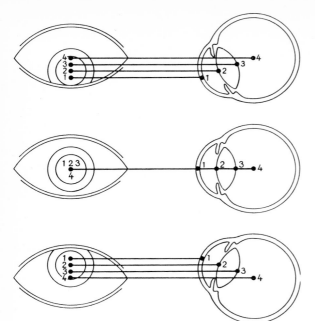

Fig. 6. Localization of opacities in the media by transillumination with the ophthalmoscope and movement of the eye (parallactic movement).

vitreous (4), will move in an opposite direction to the motion of the eye. Exactly the reserve is true for opacities lying in *front of the pupillary plane*, for instance in the cornea (1). These will move in the same direction as the eye.

b) Opacities of the Vitreous

Opacities of the vitreous appear as dots, threads or larger flakes. They float freely in the vitreous and are of varying size. They may occur in:

1. Myopia which leads to changes in the vitreous structure due to *stretching* of the eyeball and *liquefaction* of the vitreous (page 134);

2. Superior or posterior vitreous detachment: The vitreous may detach in the equatorial area or from its attachment at the optic nervehead. It will then collapse and shrink;

3. *Degenerative changes* of the vitreous structure in old age;

4. *Hemorrhages* and vascular changes in arteriosclerosis (page 104), hypertension (page 108), diabetes (page 119), retinal periphlebitis (page 100) and after contusions;

5. Due to *exudation* of cells into the vitreous in uveal diseases (iridocyclitis, choroiditis, panuveitis).

If the vitreous opacities are massive (for instance in hemophthalmus), the pupil appears on transillumination not red, but remains dark. Such conditions may lead to the formation of connective tissue strands and membranes with secondary retinal detachment (page 140).

In *synchysis scintillans* numerous small, floating, golden, glistening deposits can be seen in the liquified vitreous. These consist of cholesterol, calcium, and magnesium compounds and they rarely cause visual symptoms. The condition is nearly always unilateral.

White, glistening deposits can be seen suspended in the vitreous in the so-called *asteroid hyalitis*. These deposits resemble snowflakes and consist of calcium soaps and lipids. They occur in old patients and cause no visual disturbances.

3. Examinations with the Ophthalmoscope

a) Direct Ophthalmoscopy

Patient and physician are opposite each other. Their heads should be at about the same height. Only self-illuminating ophthalmoscopes are in use nowadays. The physician uses the right eye to examine the patient's right eye and vice versa. It is of advantage to hold the ophthalmoscope in the right hand when examining the right eye and in the left hand when examining the left eye. The index finger should always be placed on the rotating disc which enables the physician to put a lens in front of the ophthalmoscope if this should be necessary.

The examination usually begins with finding the *optic nervehead*. This oval disc is characterized by its light color which distinguishes it from the neighboring area. It lies nasally from the optic axis (fovea) (Fig. 7). In order to find the area of the optic nervehead in the patient's eye the patient has to look straight ahead and not into the ophthalmoscope. It may be of advantage to ask the patient, when his right eye is being examined, to look toward the physician's right ear.

It is usually easier for the beginner to approach the patient's eye slowly from a distance. First the pupil will appear red as in transillumination. As the physician comes closer to the patient's eye, he can look through the pupil as if viewing the ocular fundus through a keyhole (Fig. 8).

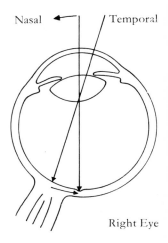

Nasal ← | / Temporal

Right Eye

Fig. 7. In order to get the optic nervehead into the center of the field, it is necessary to move the eye nasally.

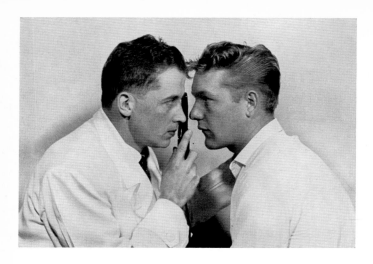

Fig. 8. Direct ophthalmoscopy.

If the patient's eye is emmetropic, the parallel rays of light will be reflected from the ocular fundus and return as parallel rays into the optical system of the physician's eye. If the physician is also emmetropic, then these parallel rays will be refracted toward his retina and a sharp image of the patient's fundus will appear in 16× magnification. Neither patient nor the physician should accommodate (Fig. 9).

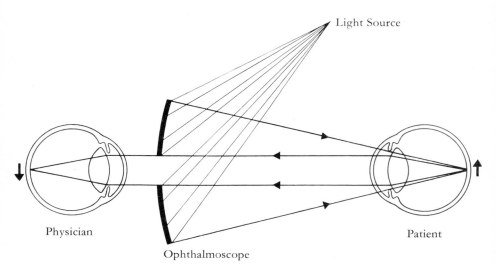

Light Source

Physician

Ophthalmoscope

Patient

Fig. 9. The course of light rays in direct ophthalmoscopy.

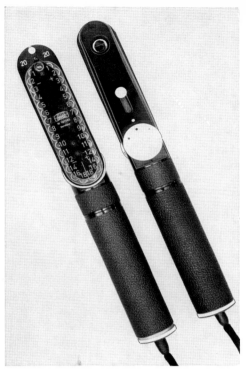

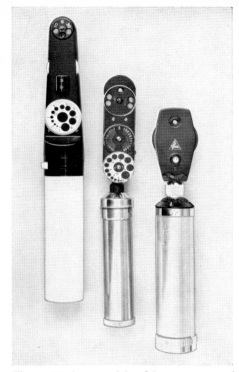

Fig. 10. Electric model of direct ophthalmoscope (Zeiss) with connection to source of
power. Left, front view; right, rear view.

Fig. 11. Various models of battery-powered
direct ophthalmoscopes.

Various models of the direct ophthalmoscope are illustrated in Figures 10
and 11.

If the patient's eye is *hyperopic*, the reflected light will leave his eye as a *divergent*
bundle of light. If the patient's eye is *myopic*, the reflected light will be *convergent*.
The physician can obtain a sharp image in these cases only by neutralizing the
patient's refractive error. Usually this is done by putting the appropriate lens into
the rotating disc of the direct ophthalmoscope. The lens necessary to view the
patient's fundus sharply will also give an indirect clue to the patient's refractive
status (see "objective refraction" page 25). This will only hold true if the physician
is emmetropic and does not use his accommodation.

An *astigmatism* (page 23) cannot be neutralized with the direct ophthalmoscope.
The retinal image remains fuzzy and minute details of the ocular fundus may be
difficult to evaluate.

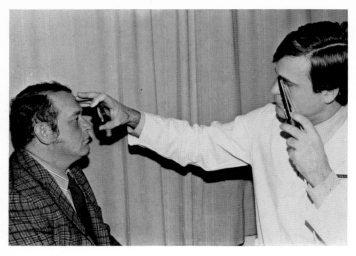

Fig. 12. Electric-powered direct ophthalmoscope.

Direct ophthalmoscopy not only permits the determination of the refractive status of the patient's eye (page 25), but also allows measuring differences in the level of the disc (page 71), the retina, and other structures of the fundus (caliber of vessels, tumors). In addition, we can determine the type of fixation used by the patient's eye by putting a cross or star into the ophthalmoscope.

b) Indirect Ophthalmoscopy

Indirect ophthalmoscopy is nowadays done with the binocular instrument which is carried on the head and is self-illuminating (SCHEPENS). In addition to the ophthalmoscope a convex lens is needed (Fig. 13).

The distance between the physician and the patient is about one-arm's length. The patient can again be examined while sitting up, but for a more thorough and careful examination it is necessary that the patient lies down. It is preferable to have the patient on a movable cart so that the patient's head can easily be approached from all sides. The lens is held in one hand at an appropriate distance from the patient's eye. The ophthalmoscope, the condensing lens and the pupil of the patient's eye have to lie on one axis. This optical system produces a virtual, inverted image of the patient's fundus at about 20 inches from the physician (Fig. 14). The physician has to accommodate on this virtual image lying in air. As the image is inverted all parts of the fundus lying below the disc appear above it and all parts temporal from the disc appear on the nasal side. Indirect ophthalmoscopy requires practice. The examiner has to learn to accommodate on the image in air, and he has to find out how to avoid annoying reflexes from the condensing lens and the cornea.

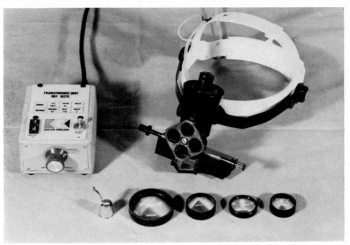

Fig. 13. Indirect binocular ophthalmoscope (Keeler) with 4 convex lenses with + 13 to + 30 diopters and a scleral depressor.

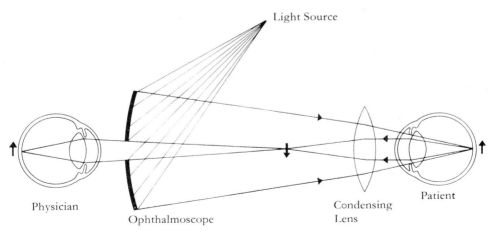

Light Source

Physician

Ophthalmoscope

Condensing Lens

Patient

Fig. 14. Course of light rays in indirect ophthalmoscopy.

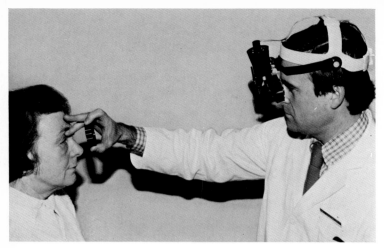

Fig. 15. Indirect ophthalmoscopy.

The technique has been well described.[1] The most frequently used condensing lens is the $+20$ D lens. The working distance of this lens is about two inches from the patient's eye. The examiner can, therefore, rest his hand on the patient's forehead. This lens gives a field of view of about $37°$ and a magnification of about $3 \times$. A good dilatation of the pupil is absolutely necessary for adequate indirect ophthalmoscopy.

In order to examine the entire periphery of the fundus, it is necessary not only for the patient to move his eyes in various directions, but also for the physician to be able to move around the patient's head (Fig. 13).

In order to see the far periphery, scleral indentation is necessary. For this purpose a thimble is used which is usually worn on the middle finger of the right hand. The tip of the depressor is applied on the skin of the eyelid over the area of the sclera to be indented. The tip of the depressor is first applied about 4 to 5 mm. behind the limbus when the patient is turning his eyes away from the examiner as far as possible. The depressor is then moved backwards slowly in the same meridian while pressure is being applied. When the depressor is about 7 mm. behind the limbus, the condensing lens is inserted into the beam of light. The condensing lens may have to be tilted according to the plane of the pupil.

Indirect ophthalmoscopy has many and great advantages. It allows the examination of the extreme periphery of the fundus even up to the plane part of the

---

[1] *Brockhurst, R. J.:* Modern Indirect Ophthalmoscopy; A. J. O. *41:* 265, 1956.

16

ciliary body. The brightness of the light is such that satisfactory examination can be obtained even when the media of the eye are cloudy. The smaller magnification produces less distortion which is optically unavoidable when looking toward the far periphery of the ocular fundus. The larger field obtained with this method allows quick checking of sick patients or small children. The binocular viewing usually gives excellent stereopsis. The advantages of direct ophthalmoscopy are the larger magnification allowing the examination of small details and the possibility of measuring fairly accurately differences in level. In this way both methods complement each other.

c) Fluorescein Angiography

Fluorescein angiography of the retinal vessels has become an important clinical examination method in ophthalmology during the last few years. This method allows an evaluation of changes in the hemodynamics of the retinal vessels, of the disturbances of vascular permeability and of pigmentation. It permits a better visualization of edema, and of degenerative and inflammatory changes of the ocular fundus. The technique is simple. Five to 10 cc. of a 5 or 10% sterile fluorescein sodium solution are injected intravenously. The ocular fundus is then examined, using appropriate filters. With specific attachments the findings can also be photographed with the fundus camera.

The dye reaches first the choroidal vessels and produces a diffuse staining of the entire ocular fundus. Shortly thereafter the dye can be seen entering the central retinal artery and its branches.

The initial stage, in which fluorescein is only found in the arterial vessels, is called the arterial phase (Fig. 16a). This is followed by the capillary phase (Fig. 16b) during which there is a fine granular fluorescence of the entire retina. Finally, there is the venous phase (Fig. 16c) with backflow of the dye through the venous vessels. This return occurs first in a lamellar form as the fluorescein-containing blood from the small vessels does not immediately mix with the blood from the other vessels. In this way the fluorescein and the normal blood run parallel. Only later will the veins be completely filled with the dye (Fig. 16d). Retinal circulation time is the interval between the entrance of the dye and the beginning of the venous backflow. This interval is shortest for the vessels which supply the macula. After about 20 seconds the dye is not visible in the retinal vessels any more. The time after the fluorescein has left the retinal vessels is called "after phase." Normal retinal vessels are not permeable for the dye and fluorescein does, therefore, not enter retinal tissues. Only in pathologic conditions will fluorescein penetrate the retina (arteriosclerotic fundus, Fig.89, or diabetic retinopathy, Fig. 105).

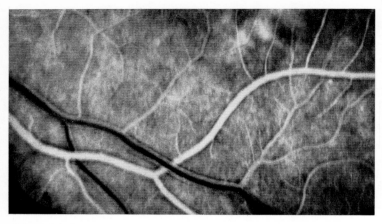

a) *Arterial phase*
The dye is primarily in the arterial vessels.

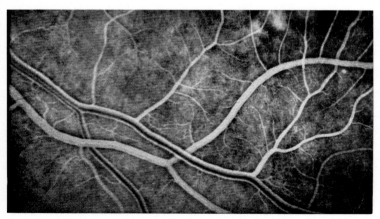

b) *Capillary phase*
There is still dye in the arterial vessels, but it begins
to fill the capillaries and the small veins. A definite
lamellar flow can be seen in the large veins.

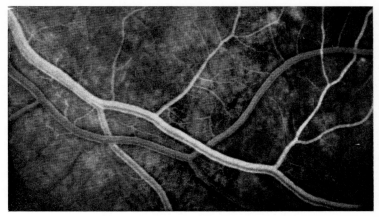

c) *Venous phase*
There is only little fluorescein left in arteries, capillaries, and venoules.
The large veins are prominently filled.

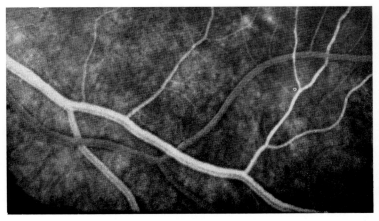

d) *Venous phase*
There is no dye left in the arteries. Only the large veins
still contain fluorescein.

Fig. 16a–d. Intravital staining of the vessels in the ocular fundus
(fluorescein angiogram). Normal eye.

4. Determination of Refraction

a) General Comments about Refraction, Anomalies of Refraction and Accommodation

The *refraction* of the eye is the relationship between the refractive power of the media (cornea, aqueous, lens and vitreous) to the lenght of the eyeball (usually 24 mm.). A beam of light which enters the eye will be refracted at the anterior and

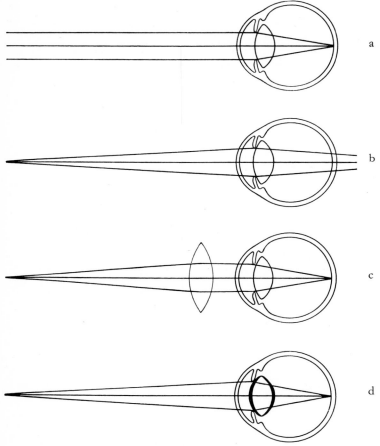

Fig. 17. Course of light rays in emmetropia.

a) Parallel bundles of light focus *on* the retina.
b) Diverging rays coming from a finite distance focus *behind* the retina.
c) Correction of near vision with a convex lens in front of the eye.
d) Correction of near vision by increasing the curvature of the lens (accommodation).

posterior surface of the cornea and at the lens. The optical factors of the eye occasionally show considerable deviations from the norm as we may expect with many other biologic factors. Such variations may be additive and may result in poor visual acuity. On the other hand, these variations may neutralize each other and good vision may still result. The normal state of refraction is called *emmetropia*.

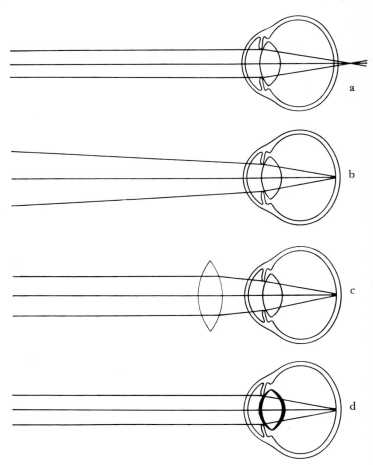

Fig. 18. Course of rays in hyperopia.

a) Parallel rays of light focus *behind* the retina.
b) Rays of light coming from the retina leave the eye as a divergent bundle.
c) Parallel rays of light can be brought to focus on the retina by a *convex lens* in front of the eye.
d) Parallel rays of light can be brought to focus on the retina by increasing the curvature of the lens (accommodation).

Such a condition exists when a parallel bundle of light rays is refracted by the eye in such a way that its focus lies on the retina (Fig. 17). Since every optical system may be reversed, we may also say that the far point of an emmetropic eye lies in the infinite, as the rays emerging from the eye run parallel.

In *anomalies of refraction* the relationship between refractive power and length of the eyeball is such that the focus of the incident light does not lie on the retina. The retina, therefore, receives a blurred image. The degree of refractive error as well as the strength of the correcting lens is expressed in diopters.

Hyperopia (far sightedness) is usually due to an abnormally short visual axis of the eye. Occasionally it is caused by the low refractive power of the media.

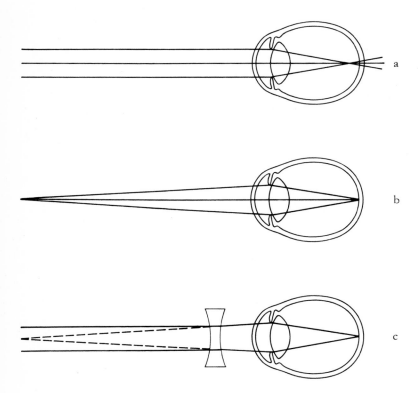

Fig. 19. Course of light in myopia.

a) Parallel rays of light focus *in front* of the retina.

b) Rays coming from the retina leave as a convergent bundle.

c) Parallel rays of light can be brought to focus on the retina by putting a *concave lens* in front of the eye.

Parallel bundles of light converge toward a focus lying behind the retina (Fig. 18a). On the other hand, rays coming from the retina leave the eye as a divergent bundle (Fig. 18b). The correction of this condition can be achieved by putting a convex (plus) lens in front of the eye (Fig. 18c). The young hyperope may compensate for his refractive error by using his accommodation (see page 21) which increases the refractive power of his eye by accentuating the curvature of his own, elastic lens (Fig. 18d).

In *myopia* (short sightedness) the visual axis is unusually long, only occasionally is the refractive power of the eye too great. At the same time there is usually a deepening of the anterior chamber and the effects of stretching can be seen in the ocular fundus (pages 61, 134). Parallel rays are refracted by the myopic eye in such a way that they focus *in front* of the retina, in the vitreous body (Fig. 19a). The image produced at the retina itself is, therefore, blurred and has hazy outlines. On the other hand, rays coming from the retina leave the eye as a convergent bundle so that the far point of the myopic eye lies at a certain distance in front of the cornea. The more pronounced the myopia, the closer will be the far point to the cornea (Fig. 19b). The myopic patient has good vision only in the area between his far and his near point and he will hold anything he wants to see clearly close to his eyes. In contrast to the young hyperope, he cannot compensate for this refractive error. Myopia is corrected with concave (minus) lenses (Fig. 19c).

In *astigmatism* there is a difference between the refractive power of the vertical and the horizontal corneal meridian. A difference of up to $1/2$ D is regarded as a "physiologic astigmatism." If the difference is larger, as for instance that produced by corneal scars, the incident rays do not meet in a focal point at all. This is, therefore, literally astigmatism, that is a point will be imaged as a line. Only rarely is astigmatism caused by differences in the curvature of the lens. The correction of this refractive error is obtained by cylindrical glasses which refract the light only in one axis, and not at all in the axis perpendicular to it.

Accommodation is the faculty of the eye to change its refractive power in order to focus a close object sharply onto the retina (Fig. 17d). The contraction of the ciliary muscle causes a relaxation of the zonule fibers (the suspensory ligament of the lens), and thereby, an increase in the curvature of the lens. The lens approaches the shape of a sphere, and during this process in this way increases its refractive power. This amplitude of accommodation depends upon the elasticity of the lens which decreases with age. The increasing sclerosis of the lens nucleus leads to a decrease in lens elasticity. The consequence is the physiologic presbyopia which occurs in an emmetrope at 40 to 45 years of age. For its correction, increasing convex lenses (reading glasses) are necessary.

In order to determine the refractive error of an eye we use subjective and objective methods of examination. Both are necessary for an exact determination.

b) Subjective Determination of Refraction

The usual method of subjectively measuring the refractive error is the *determination of visual acuity* with lenses in front of a vision chart.

The patient is seated at a distance of 6 meters from the vision chart. This distance is necessary to eliminate accommodation. Each eye is separately tested (the other eye has to be covered) as to its visual acuity for distance without correction. If the visual acuity is not normal (6/6 or, if expressed in feet, 20/20) the presence of a refractive error has to be assumed provided there are no pathologic changes in the media, the retina, the optic nerve or the higher visual pathways. We then try to obtain a normal visual acuity by putting corrective lenses in front of the patient's eye. The lens necessary to restore normal vision corresponds to the refractive error. Such *subjective* determinations of the refraction depend upon the cooperation and intelligence of the patient.

It is also possible that a certain amount of accommodation is still being used introducing a considerable error. It is, therefore, often necessary to supplement this method with an *objective* method. The latter is absolutely necessary when examining infants or small children.

c) Objective Determination of Refraction

α) Direct Ophthalmoscopy

The image produced by *direct ophthalmoscopy* will be blurred if either the physician or the patient has a refractive error (page 12). By putting a lens into the ophthalmoscope (rotating disc) the image can be sharpened and the strength of this lens corresponds then to the refractive anomaly. This measurement is fairly accurate provided neither the physician nor the patient accommodates.

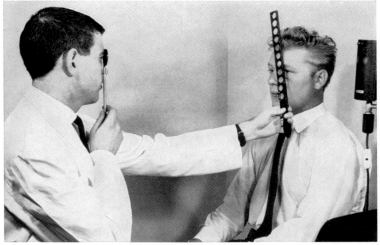

Fig. 20. Retinoscopy to determine objectively the error of refraction.

β) Retinoscopy

A more accurate way to determine objectively the refractive error is by *retinoscopy*. This is a specialized form of transillumination. A self-illuminating plane mirror is used which is perforated with a small central hole. Most modern retinoscopes have an attachment by which a streak can be produced allowing faster and more accurate determination of astigmatism (Fig. 20).

The examination has to be done in a darkened room. The physician is at a distance of approximately 1 meter from the patient's eye. The pupil of the patient has to be dilated. Cyclogyl is the drug of choice in adults, whereas in children $^1/_2$ or 1% Atropine may be necessary. The light of the retinoscope is then directed

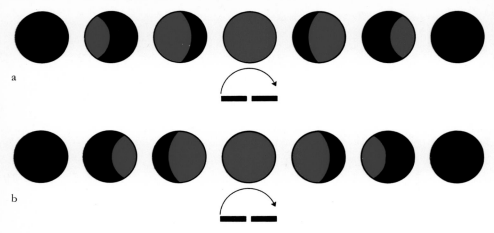

Fig. 21. The movement of light and shadows in retinoscopy rotating the mirror from the left to the right.
a) Hyperopia; b) Myopia.

toward the patient's pupil (Fig. 21). Turning the retinoscope (Fig. 22) slightly in a horizontal and vertical meridian will show the pupil light and later on completely dark. Usually a shadow will be noticed which moves in one or the other direction across the pupil.

The following possibilities may now occur:

1. The entire pupil appears bright red. Upon further rotation of the retinoscope the pupil becomes suddenly dark again without any visible movement of the shadow. In this case *emmetropia* is present (page 21).

2. When rotating the retinoscope from the left to the right, the pupil lights up first only at the left margin, whereas the rest of the pupil remains dark. With further rotation of the instrument, the light progresses toward the right beyond the center of the pupil and finally disappears at the right pupillary margin. This movement of the light is followed by a *shadow* which, therefore, also moves in the *same direction* that the instrument was rotated (Fig. 21 a). In this case *hyperopia* exists (page 22).

3. When rotating the retinoscope from left to right, the opposite area of the pupil, that is the right pupillary margin, first lights up. Upon further rotation of the instrument, the light moves toward the left beyond the pupillary center until it finally vanishes at the left pupillary margin. This movement of the light is followed by a *shadow* which also moves, therefore, in *opposite direction* to the rotation of the instrument (Fig. 21 b). In this case *myopia* exists (page 23).

The rays emerging from the eye determine the behavior of light and shadow. If the emerging rays converge to a focus in the eye of the physician, the patient's pupil will appear immediately and evenly red. If, however, the emerging rays

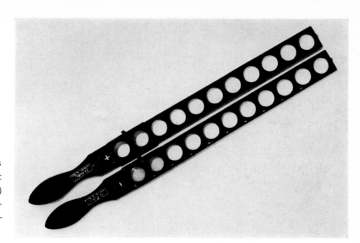

Fig. 22. Retinoscopy is performed with different strengths of plus (convex) and minus (concave) lenses for objective determination of refractions.

converge beyond the physician's eye, as is the case in *hyperopia*, light and shadow will move in the *same direction* as the retinoscope is rotated. If, however, the emerging rays are convergent, as in *myopia*, and focus onto a far point which lies between the physician and the patient, the crossing of the rays will produce a movement of the light and shadow in the *opposite direction* to the rotation of the retinoscope.

If one now wants to determine the *refractive error*, convex or concave lenses are put in front of the patient's eye until his hyperopia or myopia is neutralized. If too strong a lens is put in front of the eye, the movement of the shadow will be reversed. There will, however, be one lens which abolishes any shadow movement and at that state the pupil will momentarily appear evenly red. With this lens in front of the patient's eye the far point of the examined eye lies in the retinoscope of the physician. The lens, therefore, corresponds to the degree of the refractive error. However, 1 diopter has to be deducted from this lens as our retinoscopy is not performed from the infinite, but from a distance of 1 meter which corresponds to the focal length of a lens of 1 D strength. An *emmetropic* eye, therefore, will be neutralized with a $+1.00$ lens if the retinoscope is held at a distance of 1 meter.

Another method to determine the refraction objectively is the so-called *approximation method*. It is only a rough method and cannot be compared in accuracy with the routine retinoscopy. In the approximation method the distance of examination is varied until the neutralization point is reached. This distance can be expressed in diopters $\left(D = \dfrac{100}{d \text{ in cm}} \right)$.

Astigmatism can be accurately determined with retinoscopy. The *streak retino-scope* allows exact determination of the strength and axis of the cylinder. Cylindrical lenses, usually plus cylinders, are used to neutralize astigmatic errors.

The *refractometer* is a rarely used instrument which determines the refraction by producing a target onto the ocular fundus of the patient. It can then be determined which lens is necessary to produce a sharp image on the patient's retina.

The corneal astigmatism as well as the corneal curvature can be measured with the *keratometer*. Two targets (mires) are projected onto the anterior surface of the cornea. These targets are at a fixed distance. The distance of the catoptric images of these figures can then measured.

5. Scleral Transillumination

For this examination the eye has to be anesthetized by a drop of Ophthaine or a similar drug. The room should be dark. A *strong*, but *small source of light* is placed upon the anesthetized sclera (Fig. 24). The pupil has to be widely dilated with drops. In a normal eye the pupil appears bright red wherever light is placed on the sclera as the light passes through the coats and the interior of the eye without interference (Fig. 24a).

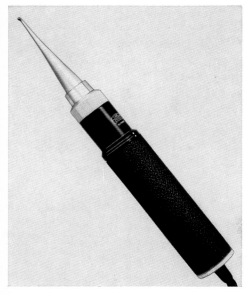

Fig. 23. One model of a transilluminating light.

A serous idiopathic retinal detachment does not present an optic interference to this transillumination. If, however, a light-absorbing tissue lies between the light source, the pupil will appear dark (Fig. 24b). Such a light-absorbing material could be a neoplasm, hemorrhage, connective tissue strands, etc. In these instances transillumination is interfered with.

This examination is of certain value in the differential diagnosis between a serous and a solid (caused by a neoplasm) retinal detachment (page 140). It also gives a certain indication as to the extent of the tumor without allowing any conclusions as to the nature of the tumor. Small tumors at the posterior pole cannot be examined in this way without opening the conjunctival sac.

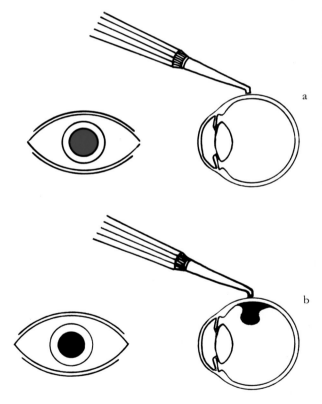

Fig. 24. The scleral transillumination.
a) In the normal eye.
b) An eye with an intraocular tumor.

I. Anatomy of the Ocular Fundus

1. The Retina

The retina is actually an exposed part of the central nervous system showing a highly differentiated structure. It is capable of visual perception and lies between the vitreous and the choroid (see page 36). In only two areas is it firmly adherent to the underlying structures: At its anterior margin (the ora serrata) and at the optic nervehead (papilla). In all other areas it is only loosely connected with the pigment epithelium.

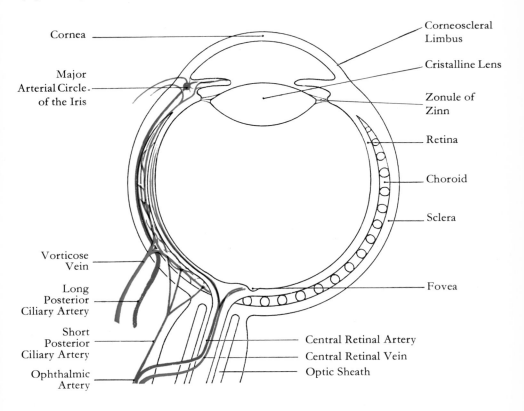

Fig. 25. Cross section through the eyeball (schematic).

The *central area of the retina* is essentially avascular. In this area the innermost retinal layers and the rods are absent. This produces a slight depression (*fovea*). This is, on the other hand, the area of highest visual acuity. It has a diameter of 1.5 mm. and contains 9,000 to 13,000 cones. These cones are especially high and narrow. They are the recipients for daylight- and color-vision.

Each cone in this area has its own bipolar and ganglion cell with corresponding nerve fiber. In this way each neural stimulation of a single visual perceptor can be transmitted to the brain as an isolated impulse. This proceeds via the so-called *papillo-macular bundle* which enters the optic nervehead on the temporal side. This bundle remains in a characteristic location in its further course to the brain.

The number of cones diminishes from the fovea toward the periphery. The number of rods, on the other hand, increases. The latter are the visual receptors of stimuli in reduced illumination. Peripheral to the fovea the 1:1 relationship between visual receptors, bipolars and ganglion cells also ceases. The border of the functioning retina is the *ora serrata*.

In pathologic conditions of the inner retinal layers the transparency of the retina decreases because of edema, hemorrhage, deposition of lipid substances, etc. In pathologic conditions of the *external* retinal layers, which occur usually as a sequel to a choroiditis (see page 158), we find destruction or proliferation of the pigment epithelium.

The *arterial blood supply* of the retina comes from the ophthalmic artery, a branch of the internal carotid. The ophthalmic artery enters the orbit through the optic foramen (Fig. 25). The central retinal artery is a branch of the ophthalmic artery. It enters, approximately 10 to 12 mm. behind the globe, next to the central retinal vein and the optic nerve. The central retinal artery branches into end-arteries within the inner retinal layers. No collaterals exist. These branches supply the second and third neurons down to the external plexiform layer. The first neuron, the visual receptor cells, is supplied by the choroidal vessels.

The *venous blood* of the retina is transported into the central retinal vein.

The *microscopic structure* of the retina resembles that of the cerebral cortex. It consists of ten layers (Fig. 26). The visual perceptor cells (neuroepithelium) lie externally, toward the sclera. The light has, therefore, to pass through the entire thickness of the retina until it reaches the rods and cones which transpose the light stimulus via chemical reactions into a nervous stimulation. This first neuron (visual receptor cells) of the visual pathway reaches to the external nuclear layer of the retina. This layer consists of the nuclei of the rods and cones. The second neuron consists of the bipolar cells. From these cells the stimulus reaches the third neuron which consists of the ganglion cells and the nerve-fiber layer. In this latter layer lie the blood vessels which are visible with the ophthalmoscope as retinal arteries and veins.

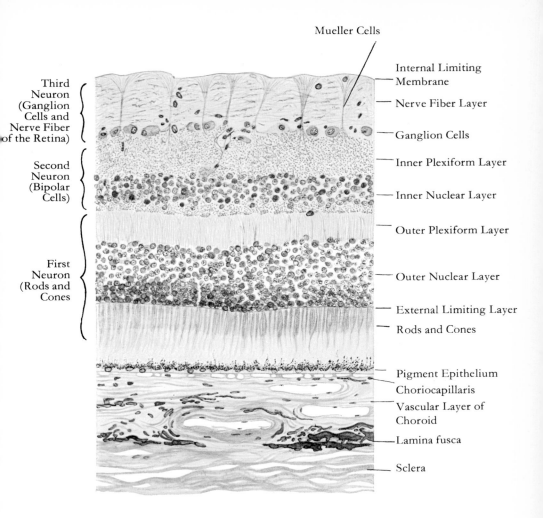

Mueller Cells

Internal Limiting Membrane

Nerve Fiber Layer

Ganglion Cells

Inner Plexiform Layer

Inner Nuclear Layer

Outer Plexiform Layer

Outer Nuclear Layer

External Limiting Layer

Rods and Cones

Pigment Epithelium

Choriocapillaris

Vascular Layer of Choroid

Lamina fusca

Sclera

Third Neuron (Ganglion Cells and Nerve Fiber of the Retina)

Second Neuron (Bipolar Cells)

First Neuron (Rods and Cones

Fig. 26. Cross section through the coats of a human eye with the layers of the retina. Hematoxylin-eosin staining, magnification 400× (from: M. WATZKA: Kurzlehrbuch der Histologie und mikroskopischen Anatomie des Menschen. 3. Aufl., S. 268. Schattauer, Stuttgart 1964).

2. The Choroid

Iris, ciliary body and choroid are also called the vascular tunic or uvea. They correspond to the pial sheath of the brain. The choroid lies between retina and sclera and is arranged in definite layers. Innermost, towards the retinal pigment epithelium, beneath Bruch's membrane (lamina vitrea) lies the choriocapillaris. This layer forms a dense net of capillaries which shows numerous anastomoses in the central area. External to this layer are the medium and large sized vessels. Outermost, beneath the sclera, lies the loose suprachoroidal tissue which resembles the arachnoid of the brain. Around these vessels is a connective tissue with collagen and elastic fibers and numerous pigmented cells (melanocytes). There are also smooth muscle fibers and a few ganglion cells. The elastic fibers lie in a regular pattern and merge anteriorly with the ciliary muscle.

The *arterial blood supply* comes mainly from the posterior ciliary arteries. The short posterior ciliary arteries pierce the sclera close to the optic nervehead, branch and supply episclera and choroid especially of the posterior pole of the fundus. A few anastomoses exist between this system and the retinal vascular system. These lie at the optic nervehead (circle of Zinn). The long arteries course without branching toward the ciliary body and the iris. The choriocapillaris supplies by diffusion the retinal pigment epithelium and the external retinal layers, especially the rods and cones.

The *venous blood* of the uvea collects in four to six vorticose veins which cross behind the equator obliquely through the sclera. These veins merge into the superior ophthalmic vein and, occasionally, also into the inferior ophthalmic vein. These pass through the superior and inferior orbital fissure into the cavernous sinus and, to a lesser extent, into the pterygoid plexus. We, therefore, can distinguish *three separate vascular systems* of the eye:

1. For the *retina:* The inner layers: Central retinal artery and vein.
   The outer layers: The short posterior ciliary arteries and the choriocapillaries.

2. For the *uvea:* Anterior and posterior ciliary arteries, vorticose veins and anterior ciliary veins.

3. For *conjunctiva* and *lids:* Internal carotid artery and ophthalmic artery, external carotid and external maxillary artery.
   Superior ophthalmic vein – temporal vein – angular vein.

3. The Optic Nerve

The optic nerve is not a peripheral nerve, but actually a *cerebral pathway* and, like the retina, a part of the central nervous system. It is composed of the neurites of the ganglion cells of the retina. The optic nervehead lies nasally from the retinal fovea and is also called *"papilla."* In this area all retinal layers are absent with the exception of the two innermost layers, namely the internal limiting membrane and the nerve-fiber layer. This is why the area of the optic nervehead is not sensitive to light, a fact which was already known to HELMHOLTZ. This area corresponds to the blind spot of the visual field, which is, however, not noticed by the patient, especially when both eyes are used together.

The optic nerve is surrounded by pia, arachnoid and dura: It has, therefore, the same sheaths as the brain. The pial sheath sends regularly arranged connective tissue septa into the optic nerve and these divide the approximately 1 million neurites into 800 fiber bundles. The anatomists, therefore, speak of an optic fascicle and not of an optic nerve.

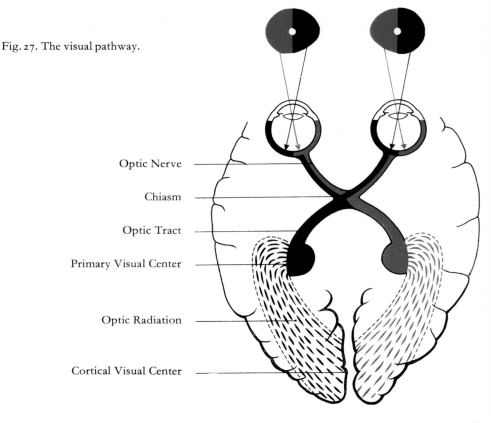

Fig. 27. The visual pathway.

Optic Nerve

Chiasm

Optic Tract

Primary Visual Center

Optic Radiation

Cortical Visual Center

At the posterior pole of the eyeball the dural sheath merges with the sclera and the pial sheath with the choroid. The space between the two sheaths is filled with cerebrospinal fluid. This space ends at the posterior pole of the eyeball. Increase in pressure of the cerebrospinal fluid leads to an ampulla-like extension of the subdural space around the optic nervehead. This produces the ophthalmoscopic picture of papilledema (see page 70) with blurred disc margins and elevation of the disc over the surounding retina.

The optic nerve is 4 to 5 cm. long extending from the eyeball to the chiasm. It consists of a intra-orbital, an intracanalicular and an intracranial part. Within the orbital adipose and connective tissue it courses in a slight S-shaped fashion enabling it to extend with the motions of the eyeball. The optic nerve leaves the orbit at the apex through the osseous optic canal situated in the smaller wing of the sphenoid bone. In this area the nerve is adherent to the bony wall and therefore especially vulnerable in head trauma.

The *visual pathway* (Fig. 27) consists of the two optic nerves converging toward the chiasm which lies on the sella turcica. Within the chiasm a semidecussation of the optic nerve-fibers takes place. The fibers coming from the nasal part of both retinas cross, whereas the fibers from the temporal parts of the retinas remain uncrossed. In this way the optic tracts are formed. The right optic tract contains the fiber bundles from the left parts of both retinas. The tracts course towards the primary visual centers in the midbrain (thalamus, external geniculate body and anterior quadrigeminal plate). Here the central neuron begins which leads via the visual radiation toward the visual center at the posterior pole of the occipital lobe above and beneath the calcarine fissure.

Pathologic changes of the ocular fundus can be expected in all processes (inflammations, tumors, trauma) affecting the optic nerve between the globe and the chiasm. Diseases of the tract, for instance inflammatory processes, neoplasms and aneurysms, may lead to a slight pallor of the optic disc. Pathologic processes of the visual radiation and of the visual cortex will not lead to changes visible in the ocular fundus.

II. The Normal Fundus

1. Color

The ocular fundus appears red when the light source in the ophthalmoscope emits primarily light of long wave lengths. The color depends upon:

1. The blood concentration in the wide, anastomosing choroidal vessels. This is the *red component*.

2. The *pigment density* of:

   a) The retinal pigment epithelium, and }
   b) the melanocytes of the choroid   } This is the *brown component*.

3. The type and intensity of the light source:

   a) The usual electric light is a red-yellow light of long wave length *(yellow component)*.

   b) A red-free light or, even better, a light with very little red component shows certain details of the retinal structure. The nerve-fiber layer and the macula are more visible. Such light can be obtained by using green filters.

Physiologic Color Variations of the Normal Ocular Fundus

A uniform red (Fig. 28), a tessellated (Fig. 30), and a poorly pigmented (Fig. 31) type of ocular fundus can be distinguished. These types depend upon the density and color of the pigment which may vary in various individuals from yellow to dark brown. The color of the fundus depends, therefore, on the pigmentation of the retinal pigment epithelium and upon the density of the choroidal melanocytes.

	Even Red Fundus	Tesselated Fundus	Blond Fundus (Albinotic)
Retinal pigment epithelium	Dense and even pigmentation	Little pigmentation	Sparse or no pigmentation
Choroidal melanocytes	Obscured	Marked pigmentation	Sparse or no pigmentation
Choroidal vessels	Obscured	Visible as red, anastomosing net; the intervascular spaces are black-brown	Visible as a red net on the yellow-white scleral background

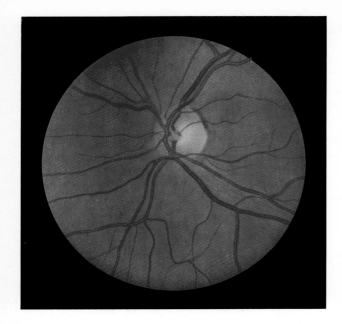

Fig. 28. Normal ocular fundus;
Even red color: In the center
is the optic nervehead with a
physiologic excavation.

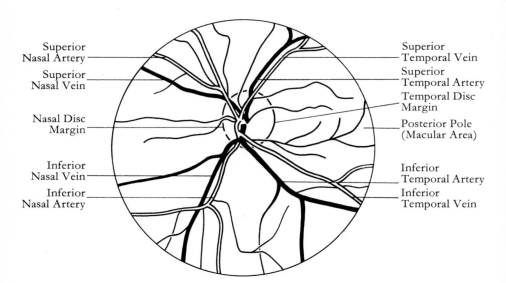

Superior
Nasal Artery

Superior
Nasal Vein

Nasal Disc
Margin

Inferior
Nasal Vein

Inferior
Nasal Artery

Superior
Temporal Vein

Superior
Temporal Artery

Temporal Disc
Margin

Posterior Pole
(Macular Area)

Inferior
Temporal Artery

Inferior
Temporal Vein

Fig. 29. Normal ocular fundus (schematic drawing of Fig. 28).

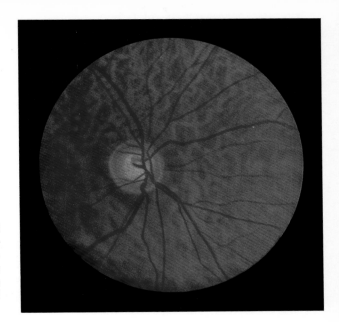

Fig. 30. Normal (tessellated) ocular fundus of a darkly pigmented patient; conspicuous contrast between the dark intervascular spaces and the light, ribbon-like choroidal vessels.

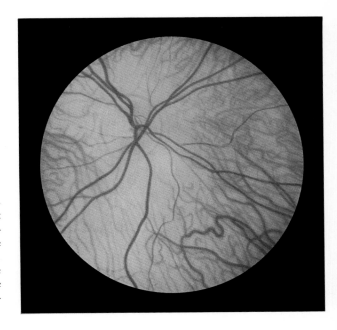

Fig. 31. Normal ocular fundus of a slightly pigmented patient (albinotic fundus). The choroidal vessels are clearly visible as an anastomosing network. The intervascular spaces are light yellow. The color of the disc is nearly that of the surrounding fundus.

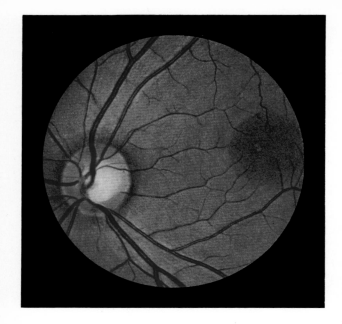

Fig. 32. Normal fundus of a Korean woman. Large physiologic excavation in the center of the optic nervehead. Marked pigmentation, especially in the area of the posterior pole (macular region).

The fundus of dark pigmented patients (Fig. 32) has an even, dark-brown color. Especially intensively colored is the posterior pole. Usually, course and arrangement of the nerve fibers are more distinctly visible than in light fundi.

The ocular fundus of an *infant* is lighter than that of an adult since the pigment concentration is slight. The choroidal vessels and the intervascular spaces are visible. Irregular pigmentation may give the fundus a piebald appearance which resembles the "pepper and salt fundus" of congenital lues (see page 160). The optic discs are less well capillarized and appear, therefore, somewhat grey or perhaps surrounded by a grey halo. This makes the differentiation from an atrophic optic nervehead occasionally difficult.

The *examination of the ocular fundus* should begin with the visualization of the *optic disc*. This area stands out because of the lighter color which differentiates it from the surrounding red (Figs. 32, 35). This should facilitate orientation. After this examination the *periphery of the fundus* should be evaluated and finally the *macular area*. This order is recommended as the examination of the macular area causes a certain amount of dazzling which may produce a constriction of the pupil if no mydriatic was given before the examination, and makes the examination of this area even more difficult.

2. The Optic Nervehead

We have to evaluate color, form, size, margin and vessels.

Color: The normal disc is slightly reddish. The temporal half is lighter than the nasal half as the number of nerve-fibers coursing over the temporal margin is smaller than the number of nerve-fibers crossing the nasal margin. In the center of the disc is usually a small white depression, the so-called *physiologic excavation* (Figs. 30, 32, 34). It is lighter than the rest of the disc. Its position, form, and size show individual variations. In its depth one may occasionally see the stippling of the cribiform plate (Fig. 33 a). A physiologic excavation never reaches the margin of the disc and this is in sharp contrast to the *pathologic*, e. g. glaucomatous, excavation (see page 82).

The presence of a large physiologic excavation or the physiologic color difference between the temporal and the nasal half of the optic disc may give rise to erroneous diagnoses of pathologic conditions (glaucomatous excavation, page 82; temporal pallor, page 78).

Form and Size: The disc is round or oval. On the temporal side there is occasionally a sickle of scleral tissue visible if choroid and pigment epithelium do not reach the disc margin. The sclera then becomes visible (temporal conus, Figs. 33 b, 49).

Margin: The margins of a normal disc are sharp. Occasionally there is a thin glial veil at the upper and lower disc margin which lies around the vessels and may simulate a certain blurriness of the margins. Also, the nasal margin may occasionally appear blurred because of the large mass of nerve-fibers crossing over this disc margin. On the temporal side we see occasionally a pigment ring or pigment conus (no clinical significance) (Fig. 35).

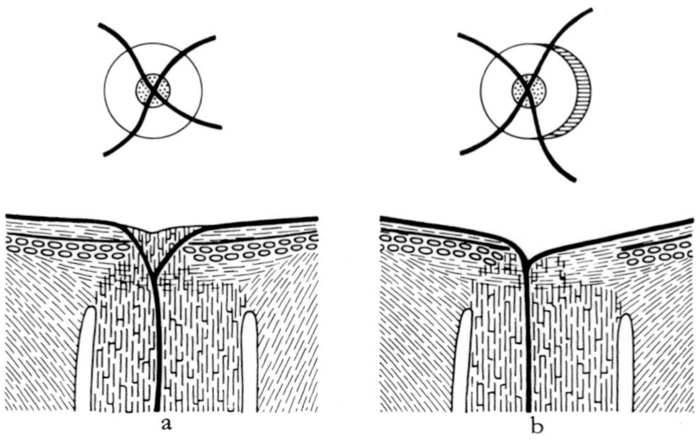

Fig. 33. a) Cross section through the optic nerve with normal disc and physiologic excavation.
b) Cross section through the optic nerve with disc, physiologic excavation and temporal conus.

Vessels: The central retinal artery and vein lie in the middle of the disc. The central retinal artery is a small artery of the muscular type. It has branches toward the circle of Zinn and it divides within the optic nervehead into four main branches. These go toward the nasal upper, the temporal upper, the nasal lower and the temporal lower periphery. The vein follows the same pattern and both vessels lie close to each other. The arterioles branch like the twigs of a tree without anastomosing with each other. Functionally we are, therefore, dealing with end-arteries. The vessels lie beneath the internal limiting membrane and supply mainly the inner retinal layers (page 36).

Appearance of the Normal Optic Nervehead (Fig. 34)

Color: Red-yellow; the red color is more pronounced on the nasal side. The temporal part may appear pale.

Form and Size: Round to oval, the diameter is 1.5 to 1.7 mm.

Margins: Sharply outlined, occasionally a pigment ring or conus (Fig. 35).

Vessels: They originate within the physiologic excavation. The arteries appear bright red and the veins dark red. There is no sheathing.

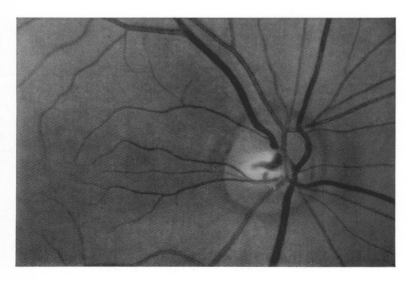

Fig. 34. Normal optic nervehead with physiologic excavation. The arterioles are bright-red and thin; the veins are dark-red and wide.

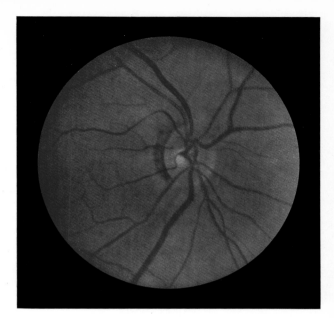

Fig. 35. Normal ocular fundus with pigment sickle on the temporal margin of the optic nervehead. The disc margins are sharp. Small physiologic excavation.

3. The Retina

The retinal *arterioles* are bright red, straight and somewhat narrower than the dark tortuous veins. There is normally a 3:2 relationship between the caliber of the veins to the caliber of the arteries. In direct illumination the vessels appear lighter in the center than in the periphery. This corresponds to the vascular lumen.

A few small branches of both temporal vessels course toward the *center of the retina* (Figs. 32, 34, 35). Occasionally, there is a large, so-called cilioretinal artery present (see page 57). A *pulsation* of the central vein is frequently visible on the disc. The presence or absence of this pulsation has no diagnostic importance. A *pulsation* of the *central artery*, on the other hand, means either that the diastolic blood pressure is extremely low or that the intraocular pressure is high.

The course of the non-myelinated *nerve fibers* is only visible when red-free illumination is used. In the center of the retina these fibers course concentrically around the fovea.

In order to evaluate the *periphery* of the retina the pupil has to be dilated with drops. In addition, the patient has to be asked to look laterally, upward and downward. The retinal periphery is normally less pigmented than the posterior pole. Near the ora serrata we frequently find pigmentary disturbances (cystoid degeneration, see page 140). This is probably due to the fact that only few vessels reach this area and the nutritional status of this part of the retina is, therefore, worse than that of the central retina.

4. The Fovea

In order to complete the examination of the ocular fundus, the *fovea centralis* has to be evaluated. It lies in the optic axis of the eye, about 3 to 4 mm. or 2 disc diameters temporal from the optic nervehead. In order to examine this area the patient has to look directly into the ophthalmoscope (Fig. 7). Many patients are dazzled by the illumination of the macular area and find this an unpleasant sensation. In addition, it will cause a marked constriction of the pupil and may leave an annoying after-image. It is, therefore, advisable to examine first the area of the optic nervehead and the retinal periphery before the macular area is evaluated. This area shows numerous individual variations which depend upon the pigmentation of the patient, his age, and the light source used. When using the normal light the macular area appears darker than the surrounding retina (Figs. 32, 36). If red-free light is used, one can see a yellowish pigmentation in the inner third of the fovea (macula *lutea*) surrounded by a faint marginal reflex. In young patients the deepest area is often characterized by the presence of a central or foveolar reflex.

The exact examination of this anatomically differentiated region (see page 34) is especially important as pathologic conditions occurring in this area (diseases of the macula) usually cause considerable visual disturbances. Their clinical appearance is manifold (see page 128).

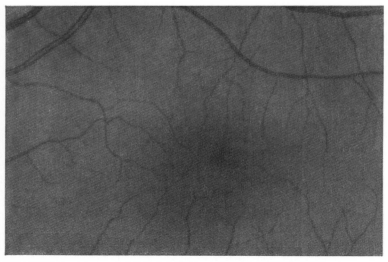

Fig. 36. Normal macular area: The yellow color of the macula lutea is visible only in red-free illumination (filter, but not with the usual light). It is not visible with the usual illumination.

5. The Choroid

The usual red color of the ocular fundus – as it appears on ophthalmoscopy – depends mainly on the vascular contents of the choroid. Details of the choroid, however, are not visible as they are obscured by the pigment epithelium in an eye of average pigmentation. Choroidal details will be visible if there is a congenital lack of pigmentation. (albinotic fundus, Fig. 31), after choroiditis (see page 153) and in degenerative processes (choroidal sclerosis, page 161; choroideremia, page 162). In these cases the ocular fundus has lost its regular brown-red color and its normal even appearance. The choroidal vessels, definite intervascular spaces and circumscribed or diffuse scars with irregular pigmentation will become visible.

Appearance of a Normal Ocular Fundus

Disc:

Color:	Red-yellow; more pronounced red on the nasal side. The temporal half may appear pale.
Form and Size:	Round to oval, diameter 1.5 to 1.7 mm.
Margins:	Sharp, occasionally a pigment ring or conus.
Vessels:	Originate within the physiologic excavation.

Retina:	Nerve-fiber layer visible only in red-free illumination.
Periphery:	Lighter than central area. Occasional irregularities of pigmentation and lighter areas visible.
Fovea:	Appears darker than the surrounding retina. Marginal reflex at the border of the macula. The yellow color visible only in red-free illumination.
Vessels:	Arteries: Light red, straight, white reflex stripes. Veins: Dark red, tortuous, pulsation. Caliber: Vein to artery = 3:2.

Choroid:

Vessels:	White, pink, yellow-white background, no reflex stripes, very tortuous, numerous anastomoses (only visible if there is dense pigmentation of the intervascular spaces, tessellated fundus, or sparse pigmentation of the retinal pigment epithelium, albinotic fundus).

III. Anomalies and Congenital Malformations

1. The Optic Disc

a) Coloboma

General

The coloboma is a unilateral, frequently hereditary malformation. It is due to an incomplete closure of the cleft of the fetal ocular cup. This cleft should close during the fifth to sixth fetal week. These defects lie according to the embryonal development of the fetal cleft nasally and down. They may affect iris, lens, retina, choroid and/or the optic nerve. A rudimentary coloboma is the so-called *inferior conus* (Fig. 37) or pit in the optic nervehead which usually lies in the lower half of the disc. Also, in addition to the coloboma, there are frequently other anomalies present, as for instance an abnormal course and position of the retinal vessels, page 57, the persistence of the artery of the primary vitreous (hyaloid artery, Fig. 42), errors of refraction (hyperopia, myopia, astigmatism), or amblyopia.

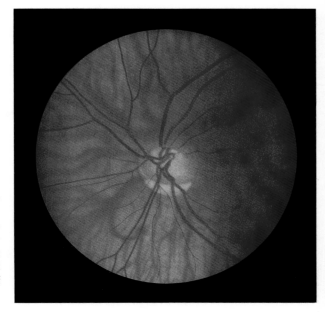

Fig. 37. Anomaly of the optic nervehead: Inferior conus (sickle-shaped atrophy of choroid and retina at the lower disc margin) and anomalous distribution of central retinal artery and vein in the center of the optic nervehead.

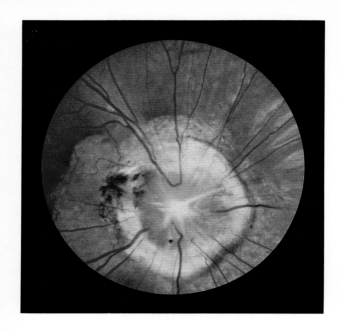

Fig. 38. Coloboma of the optic nervehead. The disc appears enlarged with a deep excavation in its center. The course of the vessels is atypical.

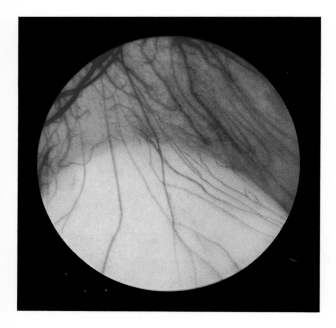

Fig. 39. Choroidal coloboma: The choroid is absent in an area which shows an arcuate margin toward the disc. In this area the white sclera is visible under the retina.

α) Coloboma of the Optic Nervehead

Colobomatous defects of the optic nervehead may be confined to the disc or may involve its surrounding. The disc may be large and deep and the central retinal vessels are absent or have an atypical course (Fig. 38). If the colobomatous changes surround the optic nervehead the disc may be nearly normal. The visual function of these eyes depends upon the extent of the malformation.

Ophthalmoscopic Finding

Disc:
Color: Grey-violet.
Form and Size: Oval, with the long axis in the horizontal meridian; deep excavation; may appear enlarged because of the coloboma.
Margins: Sharp, circumpapillary choroidal atrophy.
Vessels: Atypical course, they disappear at the disc margin into the tissue defect (the difference in the two levels can be measured in diopters) (see page 71). Because of early branching (deep bifurcations) the central retinal vessels (artery and vein) are not visible.

Differential Diagnosis

Pit of the Optic Nervehead.
Posterior Coloboma.

β) Coloboma of the Choroid

The choroidal coloboma can reach up to the disc. Occasionally it is confined to the choroid only. Then it has the shape of a parabola with its apex the disc.

Ophthalmoscopic Finding (Fig. 39)

Disc: Normal or congenital coloboma (see above).
Colobomatous area:
Color: White, as the choroid is missing and sclera becomes visible.
Form and Size: Convex margin toward disc. The width of the coloboma may vary.
Margins: Sharp, often with pigment clumps at the border (Fig. 40).
Vessels: The retinal vessels usually course over the choroidal coloboma. Choroidal vessels are totally absent in this area.

γ) Bridge Coloboma (Fig. 40)

A bridge coloboma exists when a small part of normal choroid and retina is present between the choroidal coloboma and a coloboma of the optic nerve. In such a case the two colobomatous areas are separated by a bridge.

Differential diagnosis

Old choroiditis (page 156).
Toxoplasmosis (page 158).

Pseudocoloboma is a term occasionally used for congenital toxoplasmosis of the posterior pole with large chorioretinal atrophy (Figs. 112, 140).

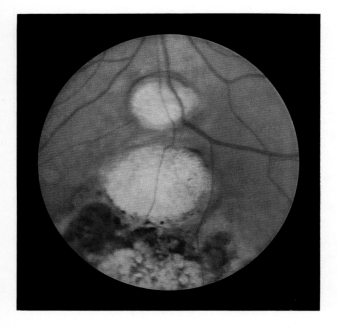

Fig. 40. Bridge coloboma. Several circumscribed defects of the choroid lie beneath the disc towards the periphery. Between them are small bridges of normal tissue.

b) Drusen of the Optic Disc

General

These are white, frequently glistening spherules which lie at the disc margin of one or both nerveheads. They occur singly or in groups. These drusen are hyaline or calcareous degenerations. Most frequently this is an innocuous anomaly. Occasionally this can be the sequel of a chronic intracranial pressure increase and papilledema or it can accompany an inflammatory process of the optic nerve. If these drusen reach unusual size, they can damage the nerve-fibers by pressure causing atrophy and thereby visual-field defects.

Ophthalmoscopic Finding (Fig. 41)

Disc:
Color: White and light.
Form and Size: Apparently increased.
Margin: Irregular, mulberry-like, sometimes slightly elevated; diamond-like.
Vessels: Unchanged.

Differential Diagnosis

Papilledema (page 70).   Secondary (post-neuritic) Optic Atrophy (page 79).

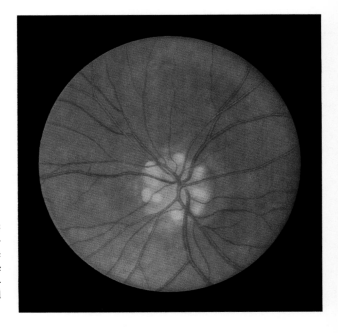

Fig. 41. Drusen of the optic nervehead: Several yellowish-white, spherical deposits are seen at the disc margin. The optic nervehead appears, there-fore, paler than normal and with blurred outlines.

c) Epipapillary Membrane

General

During fetal development the hyaloid artery courses from the disc through the vitreous toward the posterior pole of the lens. If parts of this artery persist after the termination of ocular development, its insertion on the disc (Fig. 42), or a membranous rest (epipapillary membrane, Fig. 43) may be visible on the disc. This is a harmless anomaly. The function of the eye is not involved.

Ophthalmoscopic Finding (Fig. 43)

Disc:
Color: The disc is partially or completely covered by a greyish-white, thin membrane.
Form and Size: Apparently increased.
Margins: Sharp, partially covered by the membrane.
Vessels: Unchanged; occasionally tortuous.

Differential Diagnosis

Optic Neuritis (page 67).

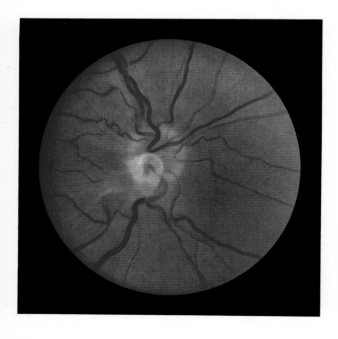

Fig. 42. Remnants of the hyaloid artery. A connective tissue remnant lies on the disc and extends like a funnel into the vitreous. In addition, there is an anomalous vascular distribution and tortuosity.

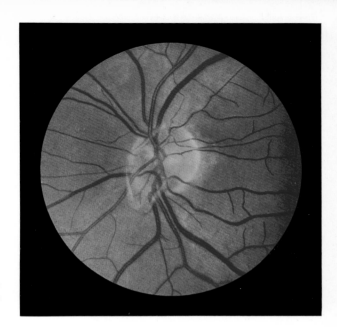

Fig. 43. Epipapillary membrane. The infero-nasal margins of the disc and the vessels are partially obscured by a membrane. The disc appears pear-shaped.

d) Myelinated Nerve-fibers

General

Normally the myelination of the fibers of the optic nerve stops at the cribriform plate. Occasionally, however, this myelinization overshoots and reaches the retina. Such myelinated retinal nerve-fibers appear as white fiber bundles with feather-like margins. Occasionally they appear as a light, flame-shaped enlargement of the disc. This is a harmless anomaly which does not affect the function of the eye.

Ophthalmoscopic Finding (Fig. 44)

Disc:
Color: Normal.
Form and Size: Flame-shaped enlargement.
Margins: In the area of the myelinated nerve-fibers somewhat irregular, in other areas sharp.
Vessels: Partly obscured, otherwise normal.
Retina: In the area of the myelinated fibers, white and glistening, otherwise normal.

Differential Diagnosis

Optic Atrophy (page 76).
Juxtapapillary Chorioretinitis (page 158).
Occlusion of a Branch of the Central Retinal Artery (page 94).

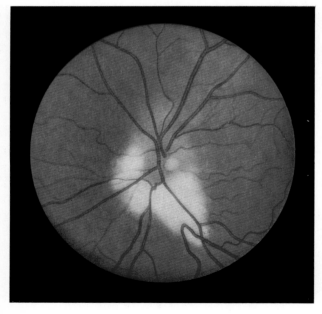

Fig. 44. Myelinated nerve-fibers at the nasal and lower disc margin. Physiologic excavation in the center of the disc.

2. Blood Vessels

a) Cilioretinal Vessels

General

Cilioretinal arteries are present in about 20% of all eyes. These are branches of the short posterior ciliary vessels or come from the circle of Zinn (page 36). They are not branches of the central retinal artery. They have a certain clinical importance in the event of a central artery occlusion (page 92). In such a case the retina supplied by the ciliary artery may retain its function. The cilioretinal artery frequently courses toward the macular area and, therefore, in such an instance central vision may be saved.

Ophthalmoscopic Finding (Fig. 45)

Disc: Color, size, and form are normal.
Vessels: In addition to the normal central vessels which come from the center of the disc, small arteries can be seen coursing in an arcuate shape over the disc margin, usually toward the temporal side and toward the macula. They have no connections with the central retinal artery.

Differential Diagnosis

Pathologic Anastomoses and Neovascularization after Occlusion of the Central Retinal Vein (page 97).

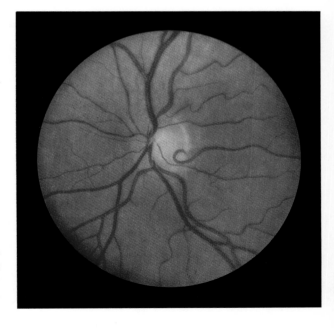

Fig. 45. Cilioretinal artery. It courses over the temporal disc margin without any connection to the central retinal artery.

b) Congenital Tortuosity

General

An increased tortuosity of all the retinal arteries and veins is found in this anomaly. This finding is usually bilateral and often associated with other anomalies of the vessels (vessel loops, cilioretinal vessels) (see page 57), colobomas or ametropias (hyperopia, astigmatism) with blurring of the disc margins (pseudopapilledema). Absent are all inflammatory changes or signs of stasis.

Ophthalmoscopic Finding (Fig. 46)

Disc:

Color, Form, and Size: Normal.

Margins: Often blurred because of the ametropia (pseudopapilledema, page 64).

Vessels: All retinal arteries and veins are markedly tortuous and dilated. They have a white, axial reflex stripe. They lie within the retinal plane. Abnormal distribution in the center of the optic nervehead.

Differential Diagnosis

Vascular changes in beginning Papilledema (page 72).
Vascular Changes in Hypertension (page 108).
Cyanosis.

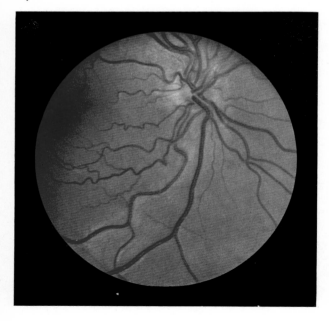

Fig. 46. Congenital tortuosity of the retinal vessels: There is increased tortuosity of all retinal vessels. The disc margins are blurred because of a hyperopic pseudopapilledema.

3. Retina and Choroid

a) Nevus

General

Choroidal nevi are usually an incidental finding since they do not produce any visual disturbance. Frequent follow-up examinations (preferably with fundus photography) are indicated to detect as early as possible an increase in size or pigmentation which could indicate a malignant degeneration.

Ophthalmoscopic Finding (Fig. 47)

Choroid: Circumscribed, well-demarcated, slate-grey pigmentation in the level of the choroid.

Differential Diagnosis

Choroidal Melanoma (page 164).
Choroidal Hemangioma.

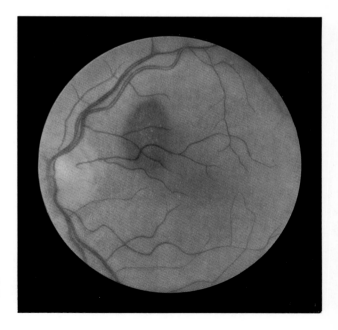

Fig. 47. Choroidal nevus; there is also a cilioretinal artery (see Fig. 45).

b) Bear Tracks of the Retina

A special kind of pigmentary anomaly are the so-called "bear tracks" or group pigmentations of the retina. These are usually confined to one segment of the fundus and consist of groups of large, brown, sharply demarcated pigmentary deposits (Fig. 48).

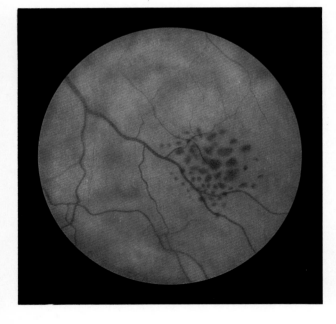

Fig. 48. Bear tracks. Group pigmentation of the retina. In addition there are several light, hazy areas due to multiple choroidal metastases from a breast carcinoma.

IV. Anomalies of Refraction

1. The Ocular Fundus in Myopia

General

Myopia is usually of the axial type (page 23). We distinguish a simple myopia, malignant myopia and excessive myopia according to the elongation of the eyeball (which may amount to several millimeters), and the stretch effect on the vitreous (page 10) and the ocular fundus. The frequent simultaneous liquefaction and opacification of the vitreous prevent a clear visualization of the fundus. In high myopia the optic nervehead courses obliquely through the sclera. In this way the retina will cover the nasal margin and give it a blurred appearance (supertraction). The pathologic thinning of sclera, choroid and retina occurs mainly at the posterior pole since the elongation occurs primarily in the longitudinal axis of the eye. These pathologic changes are especially pronounced around the disc. They may be visible only at the temporal margin (Figs. 49 a, 50). In high myopia, however, they surround the entire nervehead (Figs. 49 b, 51). Fundus changes and severity of myopia are not always in direct relationship. The marked thinning of the tissues leads to atrophic areas, to dehiscences and ruptures of Bruch's membrane producing light, net-like lines, so-called "lacquer cracks." In addition, we find irregular pigmentation along the vessels and in the macular area (Fuchs spot) (myopic macular changes, see page 134) (Fig. 117).

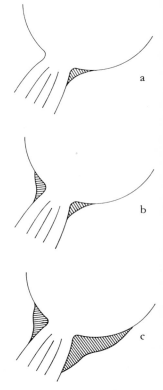

In cases of excessive myopia one sees occasionally a bulging of the circumpapillary sclera (Scarpa's staphyloma) (Fig. 49 c). The retinal vessels can be seen bending over the margin of this scleral staphyloma. In the deeper part lies the normal disc. At the same time, in other areas of the fundus there are round, oval or geographic patches of atrophic choroid and retina. These degenerative processes may lead to ruptures of small vessels and, thus, to hemorrhages and later on to pigmentary reactions.

Fig. 49. a) Temporal myopic conus. b) Peripapillary choroidal atrophy. c) Posterior staphyloma.

High myopia presents a certain disposition to retinal tears and to retinal detachment (page 140).

a) Myopic Temporal Conus (Fig. 50)

Ophthalmoscopic Finding (Fig. 50)

Disc:
Color: Normal.
Form and Size: Round, normal.
Margins: On the nasal side occasionally blurred.
Vessels: Straight.
Choroid and Retina: On the temporal side of the disc, which is closer to the longitudinal axis, there is a sickle-shaped atrophy of choroid and retina. This conus may vary in its width, form and margins. Its color is yellowish-white as the sclera shines through.

b) Circumpapillary Choroidal Atrophy

Ophthalmoscopic Finding (Fig. 51)

Disc: Normal.
Choroid and Retina: Around the disc is an area of atrophic choroid and retina which is of irregular and uneven width. The light sclera shines through. The fundus appears pale. The retinal vessels are straight. Choroidal vessels are visible.

Differential Diagnosis

If the conus is of a certain size, the evaluation of color, size and margins of the optic disc may become difficult. If the atrophy surrounds the entire disc, the optic nervehead itself will usually be evaluated as lighter than normal (atrophic) or as pathologically changed because of a blurred margin.

The myopic scleral staphyloma has to be differentiated from a coloboma (page 49) and a glaucomatous excavation (page 82). The excavation occurs within the disc itself. The staphyloma, on the other hand, affects the surrounding of the disc.

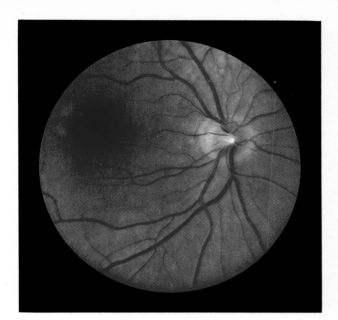

Fig. 50. Myopic temporal conus: There is a sickle-shaped atrophy of choroid and retina at the temporal disc margin. A physiologic excavation is in the center of the disc.

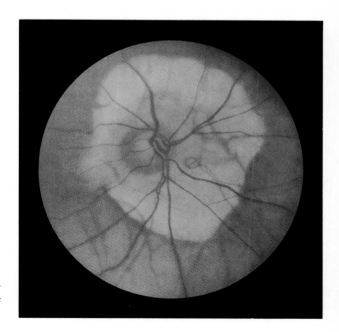

Fig. 51. Myopic circumpapillary choroidal atrophy. The disc is of normal color.

2. The Ocular Fundus in Hyperopia

General

The margins of the normal disc are always sharp, and therefore, whenever the margins appear blurred a pathologic condition should be suspected (optic neuritis, page 67, papilledema, page 70).

Occasionally, however, we find a so-called *pseudopapilledema* which is usually associated with anomalies of refraction, especially with *hyperopia* of a considerable degree. This is a harmless anomaly which is due to the fact that there is more than the usual amount of connective and glial tissue on these discs. There is also a crowding of the nerve-fibers due to the relatively narrow scleral canal of the foreshortened hyperopic eye.

In order to clarify the situation and arrive at a correct diagnosis the examination of the refractive error (page 20) is necessary.

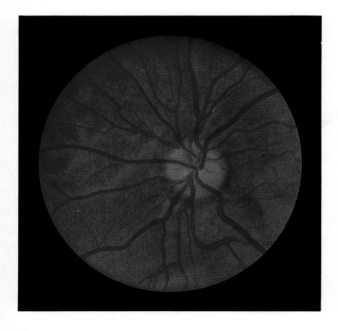

Fig. 52. Hyperopic pseudopapilledema. The disc margins are blurred all the way around.

a) Hyperopic Pseudopapilledema

Ophthalmoscopic Finding (Fig. 52)

Disc:
Color: Reddish.
Form and Size: Diameter apparently somewhat increased.
Margins: Partial or complete blurring, the disc may be slightly elevated.
Vessels: Normal caliber; however, sometimes increased tortuosity.

Differential Diagnosis

Optic Neuritis (Papillitis) (page 68).
Papilledema (page 70).

V. Diseases of the Vitreous

The vitreous is transparent, gel-like and void of any vessels or nerves. It fills the 4-cubic-centimeter cavity behind the lens and in front of the retina. It consists of 98% water. The water is bound by hyaluronic acid to the collagen fibrils which are seen electron microscopically. This collagen framework is denser toward the periphery and is separated by a basal membrane from the adjacent structures. Firm adhesions to the retina exist at the margin of the optic nervehead and at the ora serrata. During fetal development the hyaloid artery traverses the vitreous within Cloquet's canal. The artery usually disappears at term.

Remnants of this embryonal artery may persist at the disc (Figs. 42 and 43) or at the posterior lens pole (Fig. 54) as congenital anomalies.

Degenerations occur in high myopia or in senility. The vitreous then loses its consistency and its elasticity. Liquefaction sets in and with it the vitreous loses its ability to protect the retina from concussions and other mechanical insults. Vitreous opacities (page 10) are of special clinical importance. These can be examined and diagnosed by transillumination (Fig. 6), or, more accurately, with the ophthalmoscope by putting a + 10.00 lens into the disc, or on the slit lamp by using a preset lens like the Hruby lens or the 3-mirror contact lens of Goldmann. These opacities impair the transparency of the vitreous and the patient sees moving floaters and bizarre figures. Mild changes consisting of compact fibrils are seen as floaters (muscae volitantes) and are especially noticeable when the patient looks against a light background. Destruction of the vitreous and especially tears in the hyaloid membrane and detachment from the optic nervehead (posterior vitreous detachment) dispose to retinal tears and retinal detachment (page 140).

Secondary vitreous opacities and deposits occur with exudative inflammatory processes and trauma to the adjacent tissues. These can lead to loss of vision. Cellular deposits can be found with iritis and choroiditis. Hemorrhages in the vitreous are seen with retinal periphlebitis, trauma and in advanced cases of arteriosclerotic, hypertensive, or diabetic retinopathy. Retinitis proliferans may lead to connective tissue and scar formation. A vitreous abscess may be found with an intraocular foreign body or with septicemia. Occasionally, one can see a parasite (cysticercus, filaria, echinococcus) in the vitreous.

Special forms of vitreous opacities are found in external exudative retinitis of Coats' (page 144) and with retrolental fibroplasia, a condition occurring mainly in prematurely born children (page 145).

VI. Diseases of the Optic Nerve

1. Optic Neuritis

General

The cause for such an – usually unilateral – inflammation of the optic nerve can be:

Propagated from *intraocular diseases* (uveitis, juxtapapillary choroiditis).
Transmitted from *orbit* or *paranasal sinuses*.
From the *meninges* (via the vascular arachnoid and pial connective tissue).
Secondary to *toxic agents*.

The disease begins with sudden, usually severe visual disturbances due to interruption of the optic nerve-fibers. This is often associated with pain on eye movements. The course may be acute or chronic intermittent. Recovery is often complete.

The optic neuritis may be an early symptom of a demyelinating disease, which it may precede for many years. An optic neuritis which does not improve or which has several recurrences may lead to a partial or complete optic atrophy with temporal or total pallor of the disc. This is the primary optic atrophy (page 78). Pallor of the disc and visual disturbances are not always in direct relationship.

According to the *localization* of the pathologic process within the optic nerve the following types can be differentiated:

1. Retrobulbar Neuritis: This is an affection of the optic nerve behind the globe. The ocular fundus is normal in the early stages (page 68).
   The diagnosis can be made on the basis of the visual field defects (central scotoma) and on the basis of the severe reduction of visual acuity.
2. Papillitis (Intraocular Neuritis): In this neuritis, pathologic changes are visible with the ophthalmoscope (page 68).
   According to *extent* and *course* we can distinguish the following types:
a) *Retrobulbar Perineuritis:* In this instance the periphery of the optic nerve is primarily involved. This occurs, e.g., when the optic nerve is affected in the course of a severe meningitis.
b) *Interstitial Peripheral Neuritis:* This is due to an inflammation of the connective tissue septa, e.g., secondary to inflammatory processes of the paranasal sinuses or secondary to systemic infectious diseases (measles, scarlatina, diphtheria, syphilis).
c) *Axial Retrobulbar Neuritis:* This type occurs in demyelinating diseases, such as multiple sclerosis, etc. It leads to an eclectic damage of the *papillo-macular fibers* (page 34) with an early and severe decrease in visual acuity.

d) *Retrobulbar Transverse Neuritis:* In this type the entire cross section of the optic nerve is affected. This leads to complete blindness. It occurs in acute demyelinating diseases or in cases of intoxication (methyl alcohol, lead, carbon monoxide).

A *special form* of optic neuritis occurs in males during the second and third decade of life. It is a bilateral, hereditary disease which is transmitted as a sex-linked recessive character. It produces a central scotoma and leads to a yellowish optic atrophy. This is the so-called Leber's familial atrophy.

a) Retrobulbar Optic Neuritis

The disc in these instances is not involved (at least in the beginning). The severe loss of function is in marked contradistinction to the absence of ophthalmoscopic changes. This is a condition in which the patient does not see anything and the physician does not see anything either. In the later course of the disease it may, however, lead to a blurring of the disc margins and finally – as in cases of papillitis – to optic atrophy due to degeneration of the nerve-fibers. The disc becomes pale.

Ophthalmoscopic Finding: Normal in the beginning

b) Papillitis

This type of optic neuritis is characterized not only by loss of vision but also by the ophthalmoscopic picture as the process is located in the optic nervehead itself.

Ophthalmoscopic Finding (Figs. 53 and 54)

Disc:
Color: Red (hyperemic), exudation may be visible in the physiologic excavation, the cribriform plate is not visible, occasionally there are a few hemorrhages.
Form and Size: Apparently increased, the color difference between the disc and the surrounding tissue has become minimal.
Margins: Blurred, as tissue edema reaches into the surrounding retina.
Vessels: Appear prominent because of the edema. The elevation, however, is usually less than three diopters. There may be a white sheathing along the vessels close to the disc.

Differential Diagnosis

Hyperopic Pseudopapilledema (page 65).
Papilledema (page 70).
Angiospastic Retinopathy (page 112).

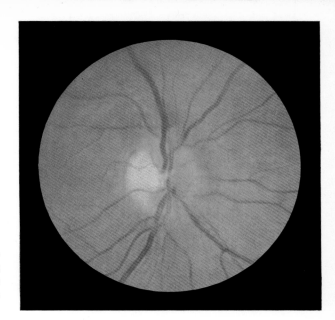

Fig. 53. Marked papillitis (intraocular optic neuritis). The disc margins are blurred, the vessels disappear partly in the peripapillary edema.

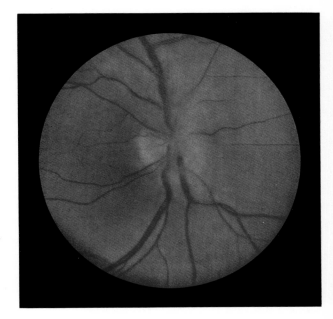

Fig. 54. Beginning papillitis (intraocular optic neuritis). The margins of the optic nervehead are slightly hazy, the disc is red and there is peripapillary edema.

69

2. Papilledema

General

Papilledema is a swelling of the optic nervehead. It has probably more diagnostic importance than any other pathologic change of the ocular fundus. Frequently it is due to a pathologic increase of the intracranial pressure and, therefore, the *bilateral* papilledema is often the *most important sign of a brain tumor*. It occurs only in about two-thirds of all brain tumors. Some intracranial tumors (like pituitary tumors) lead immediately to an optic atrophy; others cause no change in the ocular fundus whatsoever. Whether and when the papilledema will appear depends mainly on the localization of the tumor. The closer the tumor lies to the cerebrospinal fluid system (surrounding the Sylvian aqueduct and fourth ventricle, posterior fossa), the sooner will papilledema appear.

The following factors are of importance for the appearance of a papilledema: *Increase in the volume of the brain substance* due to space-consuming lesions (tumors, abscesses, hemorrhages, local or systemic edema), *changes in the pressure relationship within the various cerebrospinal fluid-containing spaces* (resistance to flow, increased production, decreased resorption), *disturbances of the cerebral vascular circulation*, of *the cerebral metabolism*, of *the permeability between vessels and central nervous system* and upon other *systemic and orbital factors*.

The increased pressure of the cerebrospinal fluid is transmitted peripherally into the sheaths of the optic nerve (Fig. 25) and into the perivascular lymph spaces of the central retinal vessels. In addition, there is a stasis of the normally centripetally flowing fluids leading to edema of the optic nerve tissue itself and, therefore, also to the papilledema.

The papilledema is among the most important signs of increased intracranial pressure (in addition to headache, nausea, etc.). It can be objectively measured. *In all cases of long lasting headache the ocular fundus has to be examined.* If papilledema is found, a general physical examination is necessary until the presumptive diagnosis of "brain tumor" can be excluded or confirmed.

A papilledema may also occur if there is a pathologic hypotony of the globe as, e. g., after a perforating injury or a fistulating operation. It also occurs with inflammations of the central nervous system (meningitis, encephalitis), in space-consuming non-neoplastic processes such as aneurysms, subarachnoidal hemorrhage or brain abscesses, in anomalies of skull growth (turricephalus) and in other diseases which may be accompanied by an increase in intracranial pressure (premature closure of the cranial sutures, cardiovascular hypertension, leukemia, tetany, etc.).

A *unilateral* papilledema is rarely seen in increased intra*cranial* pressure (about 5%). In unilateral cases we are usually dealing with a so-called "orbital" papilledema which is the consequence of an intra-*orbital* space-consuming lesion or of a compression of the optic nerve by a tumor (page 86), by hemorrhage, by edema and inflammation, by an aneurysm or thrombosis of the ophthalmic vein or of the cavernous sinus.

In the beginning the symptoms of a papilledema are minimal. The visual acuity is usually not disturbed, so that this important sign can only be diagnosed by ophthalmoscopy.

The *diagnosis* of a fully-developed papilledema (Figs. 57, 58) is not difficult. The *early stages* (Fig. 56) are, however, difficult to discern. The disc appears somewhat reddened and its margins are more or less blurred, but there may not yet be a definite elevation of the disc, nor hemorrhages.

If the papilledema persists through several weeks, an irreversible damage to the optic nerve-fibers may lead to an atrophy (Fig. 58) with visual disturbances.

Measuring the Elevation of the Disc

The elevation of the papilledema can be measured by determining the difference between the peak of the disc and the level of the surrounding retina.

The difference between the level of the elevated disc and the surrounding retina can be recognized in indirect ophthalmoscopy by the parallactic shifting of the disc margin.

An exact measurement of the elevation of the disc is possible with the direct ophthalmoscope. Such a measure is necessary for the exact evaluation of the progression or improvement of the condition (Fig. 55). We first produce a sharp image of the retina which is not affected by the edema (page 13). After this, one turns the ophthalmoscope toward the peak of the papilledema and again produces a sharp image by putting more plus lenses into the ophthalmoscope. The difference between the lenses needed for the two areas corresponds to the elevation of the disc in diopters (3 D = 1 mm.).

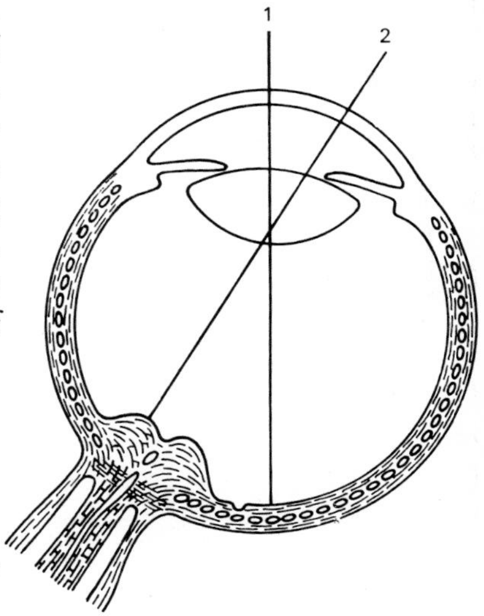

Fig. 55. Determination of the elevation of a disc by direct ophthalmoscopy.

a) Beginning Papilledema

Ophthalmoscopic Finding (Fig. 56)

Disc:
Color: Red, the capillaries on the disc are dilated.
Form and Size: Round, the diameter appears increased.
Margins: Partially or completely blurred. No or very little elevation in the early stages.
Vessels: Arteries: Normal.
                Veins: Dilated, tortuous.
Retina: Around the disc somewhat edematous, occasionally a few hemorrhages close to the disc.

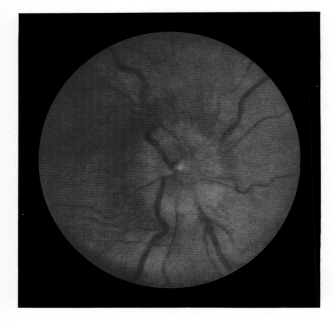

Fig. 56. Beginning papilledema: The disc is red with blurred outlines; the veins are dilated.

b) Pronounced Papilledema (Usually Bilateral)

Ophthalmoscopic Finding (Figs. 57, 58)

Disc:
Color: Greyish-red.
Form and Size: Diameter apparently increased.
Margins: Generally blurred, mushroom-like elevation toward the vitreous, well-measurable elevation.
Vessels: Are elevated over the disc, they have sheathing, the physiologic excavation has disappeared.
Arteries: Narrow, partly obscured by the edema.
Veins: Markedly dilated and tortuous, dark red, no venous pulsation.
Retina: Circumpapillary edema, radial folds, more or less numerous flame-shaped hemorrhages near the disc.

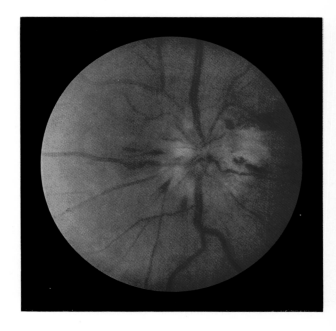

Fig. 57. Marked papilledema: Peripapillary edema, exudation into the physiologic excavation. The veins are dilated and tortuous, with flame-shaped hemorrhages at the disc margin.

73

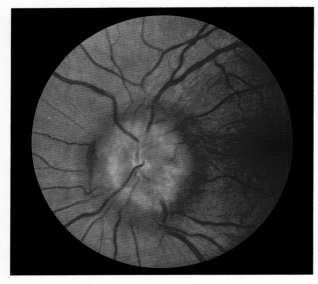

Fig. 58. Advanced papilledema. Disc margins are blurred, pale, and more elevated than normal.

Differential Diagnosis (see Table on page 75)

It is of great importance to differentiate a papilledema from other clinical pictures which look quite similar. This differentiation is especially important because of the treatment which may have to be employed. The symptoms are often non-characteristic and cannot be used in the differential diagnosis. On the other hand, the examination of the visual function should usually enable us to differentiate a papilledema from an *optic neuritis (papillitis)* (see page 68). In the *early stages* of papilledema visual function is normal except for those defects produced by other pathologic changes, such as opacities of the media, retinal changes, atrophy of the optic nerve or amblyopia. *Optic neuritis*, on the other hand, *decreases the visual acuity and the visual field early and considerably.* In the latter we are dealing with a disease of the optic nerve-fibers themselves. In addition, it should be pointed out that the elevation of the disc is, in cases of optic neuritis, usually unilateral and rarely more than three diopters in height.

In order to differentiate *papilledema* from *central vein thrombosis,* which is usually unilateral, and from an angiospastic retinopathy (usually bilateral) the *entire* fundus of both eyes has to be examined. In these two conditions we find pathologic changes of the entire vascular tree and retinal changes reaching into the periphery.

Congenital anomalies of the optic nervehead, e. g. pseudopapilledema (page 64), lack the peripapillary edema, the hemorrhages, and the exudation into the physiologic excavation. These eyes have normal veins and arteries, there is no enlargement of the blind spot, and marked hyperopia is a rather consistent finding (hyperopic pseudopapilledema).

Symptoms and Signs of Papilledema, Optic Neuritis, Occlusion of the Central Retinal Vein and Angiospastic Retinopathy

Papilledema	Optic Neuritis		Central Vein Occlusion	Angiospastic Retinopathy
Headache Vertigo Vomiting	Visual Disturbances Pain on Eye Movements	SYMPTOMS	Unilateral Loss of Vision	Headache
		SIGNS *Ocular Fundus*		
Usually bilateral	Usually unilateral	Localization	Unilateral	Bilateral
Blurred, elevated Flame-shaped hemorrhages	Blurred Not elevated	Disc	Blurred	Blurred, slightly elevated
Sheathing		Retinal Vessels	*Bilateral attenuation of arterioles, dilated veins, tortuous, A. V. nicking*	
Circumpapillary edema	Circumpapillary edema	Retina	*Unilateral:* Massive hemorrhages reaching into periphery, later white areas of degeneration	*Bilateral:* Hemorrhages
Folds Later exudates				Circumpapillary ischemia Macular star
		Function		
Normal in early stages	Immediately decreased	Visual acuity	Decreased	Occasionally decreased
Constricted (corresponding to damage to visual pathway)	Constricted	Visual fields	Normal	Usually normal
Enlarged	Enlarged	Blindspot	Usually normal	Normal
Normal	Decreased	Light sense	Normal	Normal
		General		
Normal	Normal	Vascular Status	Often hypertension or arteriosclerosis	Hypertension
Normal	Normal	Kidney Function	Decreased	Decreased

3. Optic Atrophy

General

Various pathologic processes (traumas, toxins, inflammation, tumors) may in the course of weeks or months lead to irreversible damage of the optic nerve and, therefore, to its *atrophy*. The disc will appear pale and grey due to the disappearance of optic nerve-fibers, atrophy of the capillaries, proliferation of glial and connective tissue. If the tissue in front of the cribriform plate decreases, an atrophic excavation will appear and the cribriform plate itself will become visible in it as a stippling pattern. According to the extent of the damage either a partial (usually temporal) or a complete optic atrophy (see below) will result. This is usually associated with a more or less pronounced disturbance of visual function (decreased acuity, constriction of visual fields). It has to be emphasized, however, that the color of the disc alone does not allow a definite conclusion as to the visual function. Even in cases of pronounced optic atrophy, the vision may still be quite satisfactory.

In order to diagnose an affection of the optic nerve not only the optic nerve-head has to be examined, but the history has to be evaluated and the entire fundus and the retinal vessels have to be observed. In addition, visual acuity, visual fields, and, occasionally, dark adaptation have to be determined. In many cases, a neurologic and neuroradiologic examination is needed.

a) Complete Primary Optic Atrophy

A primary atrophy may be found after a *trauma* (fracture of the base of the skull) which has damaged the optic nerve. It is important to know that immediately after the injury the disc may appear completely normal though the patient is already totally blind on this side (with lack of direct pupillary reaction). It takes some time before the degeneration of the optic nerve-fibers becomes apparent and only after three to four weeks will a pallor of the disc appear. This atrophy may involve the *entire* disc (*total atrophy*) or only *part of it*, for instance the temporal sector (see page 78).

An *intrasellar tumor* (pituitary adenoma) may also lead to a primary atrophy by compression of the optic nerve. In these cases we find usually characteristic, often bitemporal visual field defects which are indicative of a chiasmal lesion (Fig. 27).

Arteriosclerosis of the vessels of the optic nerve may first lead to a vascular papilledema (Fig. 90) and then to a primary (vascular) atrophy (opticomalacia) (Fig. 91). In these cases we usually find similar sclerotic changes of the retinal vessels (page 104). Occasionally, this type of optic atrophy, leading to a sudden loss of vision, is caused by a *temporal arteritis* (giant cell arteritis) (see page 116).

Several *toxic substances*, such as nicotine, lead, arsenic, methyl alcohol, carbon dioxide, quinine and thallium, and *diseases of the central nervous system* (such as tabes dorsalis and general paresis), as well as *severe blood loss* may lead to a primary, usually bilateral, optic atrophy.

Ophthalmoscopic Finding (Fig. 59)

Disc:
Color: Chalky-white or porcelain-white.
Form and Size: Normal.
Margins: Normal.
Vessels: Normal to attenuated.

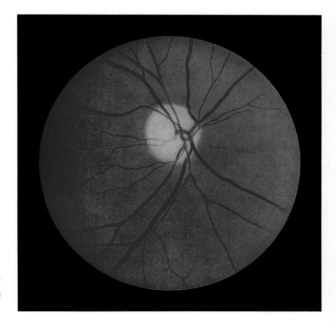

Fig. 59. Complete primary optic atrophy. Disc is white and sharply outlined.

b) Partial Primary Optic Atrophy (Temporal Pallor)

A partial primary optic atrophy represents itself usually as a temporal pallor. It is the end-result of a damage to the papillo-macular bundle of the optic nerve-fibers. This bundle courses over the temporal half of the disc and runs further centrally in the middle of the optic nerve. This fiber bundle, which transmits impulses from the area of highest visual acuity, is especially vulnerable to attacks of demyelinating diseases, optic neuritis due to paranasal sinusitis or intoxications (see above).

Frequently the temporal pallor is but the initial stage of a complete optic atrophy.

Ophthalmoscopic Finding (Fig. 60)

Disc:
Color: The *temporal* half is paler than normal; the nasal half appears normal.
Form and Size: Normal.
Margins: Sharply outlined.
Vessels: Normal.

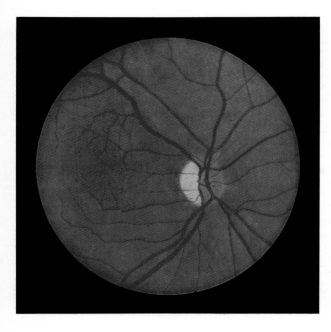

Fig. 60. Partial primary optic atrophy (temporal pallor).

c) Post-Neuritic Optic Atrophy

The neuritic optic atrophy is the end-result of a long lasting inflammation and edema of the optic nervehead. The more pronounced the swelling, the more marked will be the blurriness of the disc margin. If the optic neuritis is a *retro*bulbar one, that means *distant* from the optic nervehead, the end-result will be a primary atrophy with sharply demarcated disc margins.

Ophthalmoscopic Finding (Fig. 61)

Disc:
Color: Chalky to grey-white, inflammatory tissue in the physiologic excavation.
Form and Size: Apparently increased.
Margins: Blurred, occasionally slightly elevated.
Vessels: Tortuous, grey-white sheathing adjacent to the disc.

A long lasting papilledema may produce an ophthalmoscopic picture quite similar to the post-neuritic optic atrophy *(atrophy after papilledema)* (Figs. 62, 63).

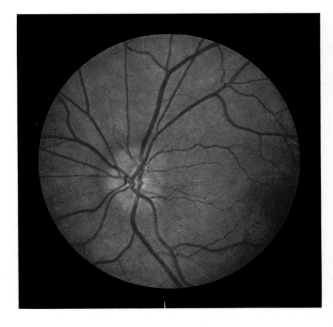

Fig. 61. Post-neuritic optic atrophy: The disc is pale and the margins are blurred.

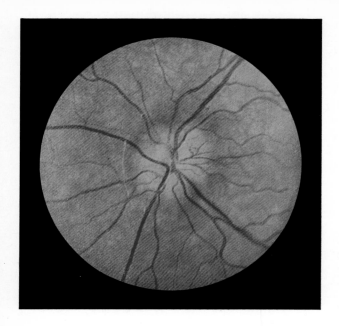

Fig. 62. Beginning optic atrophy after papilledema. The disc is pale with blurred outlines. The veins are dilated. Small hemorrhages are below the disc.

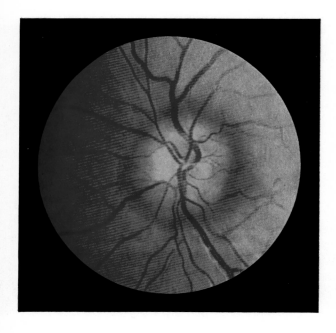

Fig. 63. Optic atrophy after papilledema: Disc is pale with blurred margins.

d) Retinal Optic Atrophy

A retinal optic atrophy is the consequence of an ascending degeneration of the peripheral neuron. This is due to an extensive disease of the retina with destruction of the ganglion cells and the nerve-fiber layer. This occurs, e.g., in pigmentary degenerations of the retina (page 138), familial amaurotic idiocy (page 138), occlusion of the central retinal artery (page 92), disseminated chorioretinitis (page 153), quinine intoxication, etc.

In cases of pigmentary degeneration of the retina, the optic atrophy is characterized by the waxy-yellow color with occasionally slightly blurred margins and highly attenuated vessels. In the retinal periphery the bone-corpuscle-like pigmentations are visible (Figs. 64 and 120).

Ophthalmoscopic Finding (Fig. 64)

Disc:
Color: Waxy-yellow.
Form and Size: Normal.
Margins: Sharply outlined, occasionally slightly blurred.
Vessels: Arterioles and veins extremely attenuated.

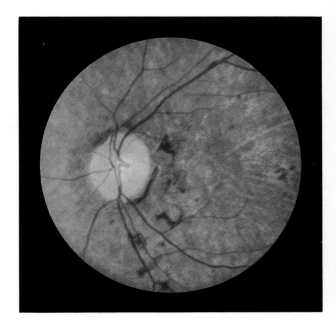

Fig. 64. Retinal (waxy-yellow) optic atrophy with pigmentary degeneration of the retina. Blood vessels are thread-like.

e) Glaucomatous Optic Atrophy

A glaucomatous optic atrophy is the end-result of a chronic glaucoma. Because of the pathologic increase of the intraocular pressure, the disc, which is the weakest part of the ocular coats, will show a bulging backward in the center (glaucomatous excavation). This is accompanied by a displacement of the retinal vessels towards the nasal side, by a bending of the vessels over the disc margin, and finally, by an irreversible pressure-damage of the nerve-fibers leading to optic atrophy. The difference between the level of the disc margin and the excavated center of the nervehead can be recognized in direct ophthalmoscopy by the parallactic shift of the central retinal vessels (Fig. 65). In the depth of the excavation the stippling of the cribriform plate can be seen. Around the disc is occasionally a light halo. This glaucomatous halo corresponds to an atrophy of the circumpapillary choroid.

Ophthalmoscopic Finding (Figs. 66, 67)

Disc:
Color: White, greyish-green; cribriform plate visible.
Form and Size: Normal, occasionally a circumpapillary glaucomatous halo.
Margins: Sharp.
Vessels: Marked bending of the vessels at the disc margin, nasal shift of the entire vascular tree. The vessels dip into a deep excavation.

Differential Diagnosis

Physiologic (Figs. 32, 34) and Senile Excavations.

(The intraocular pressure has to be measured! Determine the visual field and the blind spot.)

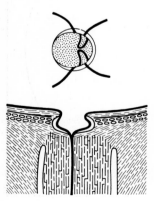

Fig. 65. Transverse section through the optic nerve and disc with large glaucomatous excavation.

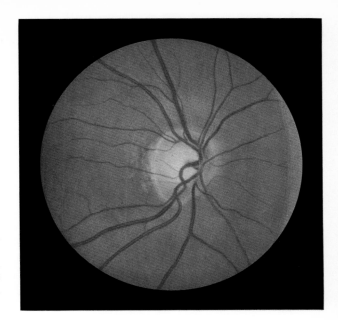

Fig. 66. Beginning glaucomatous excavation. The central part of the disc is excavated. The vascular tree is pushed nasally and there is a slight bending of the retinal vessels over the disc margin.

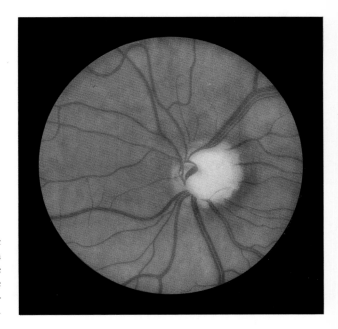

Fig. 67. Glaucomatous optic atrophy: The disc is pale with a large excavation reaching the disc margin. The vessels are pushed nasally and show a definite step at the disc margin.

4. The Foster-Kennedy Syndrome

General

The Foster-Kennedy syndrome is most often found with tumors of the anterior cerebral fossa (tumors of the frontal lobe, meningiomas of the olfactory groove).

In the initial stages we find a *primary optic atrophy* on the side of the tumor due to compression of the intracranial optic nerve. Later on, the increase in the size of the tumor will lead to an increase in intracranial pressure and, therefore, to a *papilledema* on the contralateral side, while the atrophic, gliomatous nervehead cannot become edematous any more.

Ophthalmoscopic Finding (Figs. 68, 69)

Disc: On the one side, white and sharply outlined. On the other side, red with blurred disc margins, mushroom-like elevation.

Vessels: On one side, normal. On the other side, tortuous, elevated over the disc margin, dilated veins.

Retina: One side normal; on the other side peripapillary edema and hemorrhages.

Differential Diagnosis

Optic Neuritis on the second eye (page 67).

Pseudo-Foster-Kennedy Syndrome: Vascular optic atrophy on one side, vascular pseudopapillitis on the other side.

Figs. 68 and 69. Foster-Kennedy syndrome.

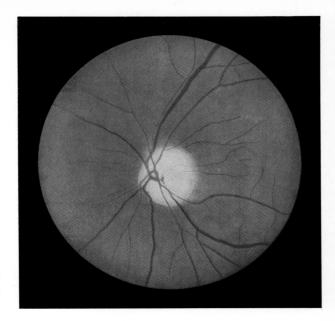

Fig. 68. Left eye: Primary optic atrophy, disc white, outlines sharp, vessels normal.

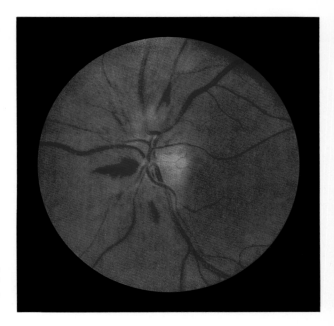

Fig. 69. Right eye: Papilledema, disc margins blurred, peripapillary hemorrhages above, veins dilated, disc elevated.

5. Tumors

General

Tumors of the optic nerve and its sheaths (glioma and meningioma) occur often in the intracanalicular and intra-orbital part. They lead to an early decrease of visual acuity and exophthalmos. If the intracanalicular part is involved, the optic foramen will become enlarged (this may be visible on appropriate x-ray pictures). These tumors occur usually in children and young adults. These tumors have a low malignancy and grow very slowly.

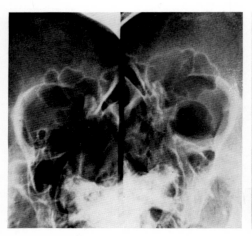

Fig. 70. X-ray picture of the orbit with glioma of the left optic nerve. The right optic canal is of normal width. The left is dilated.

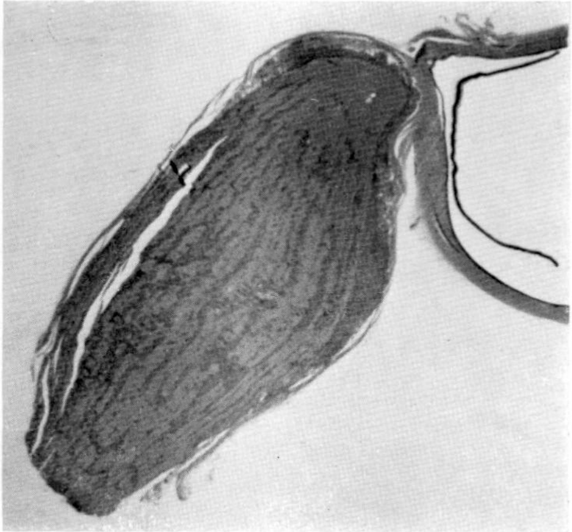

Fig. 71. Glioma of the optic nerve.

Ophthalmoscopic Finding

According to the localization and growth of the tumor we find a primary optic atrophy (page 76) or, if the tumor leads to an increase in orbital volume, a unilateral (orbital) papilledema (page 70).

Differential Diagnosis

Optic atrophy of different etiology (page 76).
Papilledema with increased intracranial pressure (usually bilateral) (page 70).

6. Injuries

Injuries of the orbit by bullets, cuts, blunt trauma, with fractures of the base of the skull, or severe contusions can damage the optic nerve by compression, hematoma formation or evulsion from the scleral canal. In the latter cases we find instead of the optic nervehead a deep hole unless extensive hemorrhages prevent a visualization of the fundus.

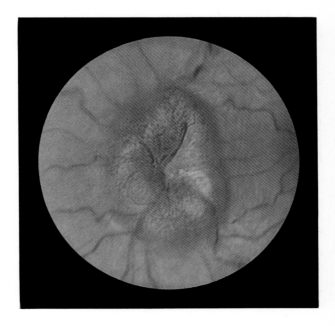

Fig. 72. Hematoma of the sheaths of the optic nerve.

Subdural hematomas or fractures of the base of the skull may produce *hemorrhages* into the sheaths of the optic nerve. If this condition causes any ophthalmoscopic changes, they may resemble the picture of an optic neuritis or papilledema. The disc margins are blurred, the veins dilated, and retinal hemorrhages are present.

The most frequent traumatic damage to the optic nerve is caused by a fracture within the osseous optic canal. In this area the nerve is adherent to the bony wall (page 38) and slight dislocations of the fragments may lead to compression, distortion or cuts of the optic nerve. The ophthalmoscopic changes of the nervehead are in the early stages minimal, but the dilated pupil which does not react to light should be an indication of the severe damage. First signs of an optic atrophy will be visible after approximately three weeks (page 76).

VII. Diseases of the Retina

1. General Remarks about Retinitis and Retinopathy

The term "retinitis" is used not only for true *inflammatory* conditions of the retina, as for instance in septicemia (see page 126), but occasionally also for *degenerative* diseases as they occur in cardiovascular diseases (arteriosclerosis, hypertension), kidney diseases (nephrosclerosis, eclampsia), metabolic disturbances (diabetes), and blood dyscrasias (anemia, leukemia, macroglobulinemia). The modern usage, however, confines the term "retinitis" only to the truly inflammatory conditions, whereas all others are called *"retinopathy."*

The ophthalmoscopic examination of the ocular fundus allows a direct observation of the retinal blood vessels. The ophthalmoscopic findings may allow certain conclusions as to the vascular status of the entire body and it is, therefore, most valuable for the evaluation of numerous systemic diseases.

First of all we are interested in the status of the *vessels:*

> The width of the vessels,
> the vascular reflexes,
> the thickness of the vascular wall,
> the course of the vessels and
> the relationship between arteriolar and venous caliber.

In addition, we may see the sequelae of an acute or chronic *vascular occlusion.* These are so obvious because the retinal arterioles are end-arterioles.

It has to be kept in mind that the retina is supplied by two vascular networks, the central retinal artery and the vascular network of the choroid (page 36). Retinal and choroidal vessels may not be affected in the same way and to the same extent. The resulting damage and ophthalmoscopic picture depend, therefore, upon the vascular system affected.

The ophthalmoscopic picture of a retinal disease is mainly characterized by:
1. Small, brownish-red hemorrhages.
2. Usually small retinal deposits, lying isolated or in groups.

These small deposits occur not only in acute inflammatory and edematous processes, but also as scars of retinal tissue following destruction of nervous substance. Contrary to the large, frequently geographic, choroidal atrophic areas the *retinal deposits are usually small.*

The function of the eye will suffer depending upon the extent and localization of the retinal changes. Small deposits in the macular area will be more noticeable than large foci or hemorrhages in the periphery.

Ophthalmoscopic Finding

Retina: The vascular changes lead to brownish-red, dot-like or flame-shaped hemorrhages which lie in the superficial layers. Occasionally, there are large hemorrhages in the deep retinal layers (see below).

Retinal Deposits:

Color: Porcelain-white or yellow, glistening.

Form and Size: Initially small; frequently they lie close to a retinal vessel, or in groups between the disc and the macula.

Margins: The fresh deposits are fluffy (cotton-wool patches). Older deposits are sharply outlined.

2. Retinal Hemorrhages

General

Retinal hemorrhages occur in degenerative (arteriosclerosis, hypertension, myopia), inflammatory (periphlebitis), and toxic vascular diseases. They also can be seen in blood dyscrasias (leukemia, purpura), in metabolic disease (diabetes), and after trauma.

If at the same time a vitreous hemorrhage is present (page 10), the accurate examination of the ocular fundus, of the blood vessels, and of the leaking vessel may be extremely difficult. A clear ophthalmoscopic picture then cannot be obtained and the absorption of the vitreous hemorrhage may take time.

Ophthalmoscopic Finding

We distinguish according to localization:

1. *Preretinal hemorrhage* (between retina and vitreous), light red, boat-shaped with a convex margin downward. In the standing patient there is a definite horizontal level. The internal limiting membrane is not broken. A sedimentation of the blood may be visible in the hemorrhage. The hemorrhage obscures the retinal vessels (Fig. 73).

2. *Intraretinal hemorrhages* (flame-shaped in the inner retinal layers), brownish-red, blurred outlines, the retinal vessels are partially obscured (Fig. 74). These hemorrhages occur in diabetic retinopathy, central vein occlusion, etc.

3. *Subretinal hemorrhages*, dark grey-violet-black, disc-shaped. The retinal vessels cross over them (Fig. 74).

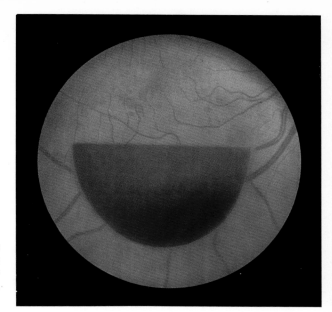

Fig. 73. Preretinal hemorrhage with horizontal level. Because of sedimentation the lower part of the hemorrhage appears darker than the upper part.

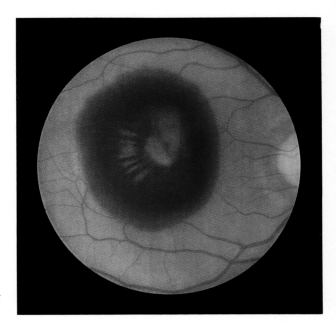

Fig. 74. Partly intra- and partly subretinal hemorrhage.

3. Central Artery Occlusion

General

This condition, originally called "embolism" by A. von Graefe (1869), is only rarely a true embolus, though this may occur in endocarditis, thromboangiitis, or with fat or air emboli. The cause for the occlusion is more often a disease of the vascular walls (thrombosis). This may be due to arteriosclerosis or hypertension or, in young patients, to a vascular spasm. Since the central retinal artery is an end-artery and no collaterals can develop, the occlusion of this vessel will produce a very sudden, unilateral, severe loss of vision (Differential Diagnosis: Optic Neuritis, page 67). Visible then is the extensive ischemia of the retina with markedly attenuated vessels. This leads within a few minutes to an intensive edema of the inner retinal layers which prevents the visualization of the choroid through the opaque retina. Only in the *macular area* will the edema be minimal as here the inner retinal layers are thin or absent. In this area, therefore, the choroid will still shine through as a red disc (cherry-red spot). This will often lead to a retinal optic atrophy (page 81). If a cilioretinal artery is present (page 57), the macula may be saved since this artery comes from the ciliary system (Fig. 76). This may lead to some salvage of central vision. In general the prognosis is poor as the treatment would have to be initiated within hours, before irreversible damage has occurred.

The occlusion may occur in the stem of the central artery or in one of the branches.

a) Central Artery Occlusion

Ophthalmoscopic Finding (Figs. 75, 76)

Disc:	Normal color, blurred margins.
Vessels:	Arteries: Extremely attenuated, collapsed, bloodless; occasionally a fine and interrupted blood flow (boxcar phenomenon).
	Veins: Usually unchanged.
Retina:	Ischemic; milky-grey to white, the macular area appears red; occasionally flame-shaped hemorrhages.
Choroid:	Invisible because of retinal edema.

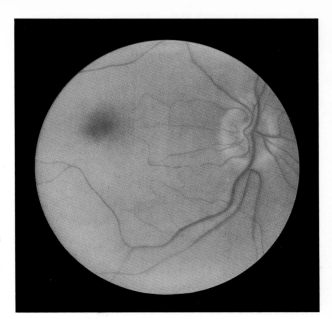

Fig. 75. Occlusion of the central retinal artery (embolism): Extensive ischemia of the retina, "cherry-red spot" in the macular area, because the choroid shines through.

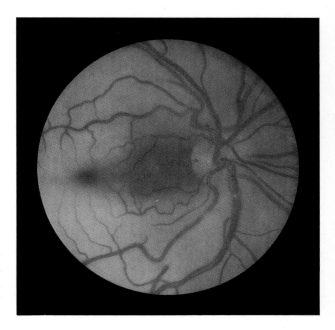

Fig. 76. Central retinal artery occlusion (embolism): The ischemia between disc and macula is not so pronounced here as in Figure 75 due to the presence of a cilioretinal artery.

b) Occlusion of a Branch of the Central Retinal Artery

Ophthalmoscopic Finding (Figs. 78, 79)

If not all, but only one or two branches are occluded, the visual disturbances are not so dramatic. The above-described objective changes (attenuation of arterioles, ischemia of retina and edema) are confined to the area supplied by the affected branch. If the branch occlusion lies close to the disc, the margin of this sector will appear blurred, but in all other sectors the margin will remain sharp. The border between the ischemic and the normal retinal areas is a sharp one. The history often reveals preceding transient (ischemic) episode of obscuration.

Occasionally one sees light, partly glistening deposits, so-called plaques (Fig. 79) at an arteriolar branching or vascular crossing. These plaques frequently lie at the beginning of the ischemic retinal sector and have been interpreted as emboli. Against this assumption, however, is the fact that the plaques may appear larger than the caliber of the vessels so that they are probably only a reflex phenomenon due to the pathologic changes in the vessel wall.

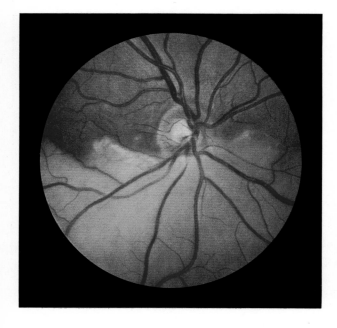

Fig. 77. Occlusion (embolism) of both lower branches of the central retinal artery. The lower part of the retina which is supplied by these two arteries is ischemic. The upper part of the retina is well vascularized.

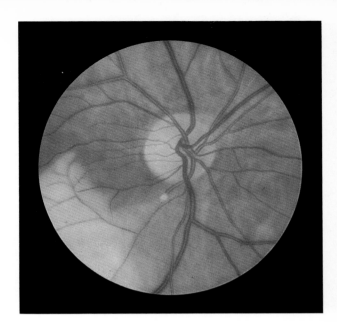

Fig. 78. Occlusion of a branch of the central retinal artery (embolism): The retinal ischemia is present only in the lower temporal segment supplied by the inferior temporal artery.

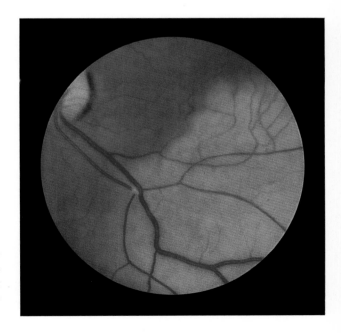

Fig. 79. Occlusion of a branch of the central retinal artery (embolism): The lower temporal periphery is affected. At a vascular branching and crossing is a so-called plaque.

4. Central Vein Occlusion

General

J. VON MICHEL (1878) called the occlusion of the central vein a "central vein thrombosis." In young patients these are probably caused by hemodynamic factors and neurovascular disturbances. In older patients they occur with systemic arteriosclerosis, hypertension, or diabetic vascular changes. As in cases of arterial occlusion, the changes of the *arterial wall* is the primary cause here. Usually, the vein is compressed by the hardened artery. This occurs at the cribriform plate because, in this so-called "cribriform plate tunnel" (R. THIEL), artery and vein lie close together and are surrounded by a common connective tissue sheath. The occlusion leads to a maximal stasis with dilatation and tortuosity of all the retinal veins (prethrombosis). Numerous hemorrhages finally occur around the vessels in the inner retinal layers reaching the periphery. With time, these hemorrhages are absorbed or transformed into connective tissue and glial scars. This leads to the appearance of light, degenerative patches in the retina, to the formation of collaterals and secondary anastomoses and to newly-formed blood vessels which may lie on the disc (Fig. 82), but also may be found in the periphery.

The visual loss (nearly always unilateral) is not as pronounced as in an arterial occlusion neither does it occur as abruptly. It depends upon the number and

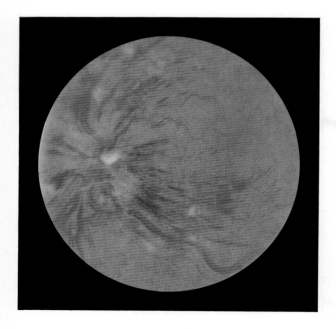

Fig. 80. Subacute occlusion of the central retinal vein (thrombosis): The veins are dilated and there are numerous retinal hemorrhages and degenerative foci over the entire fundus. The disc is hyperemic.

localization of the retinal hemorrhages. Here also, we distinguish between an occlusion of the central retinal vein and one or several of its branches, depending on where the occlusion occurs. The prognosis is better than in eyes with central retinal artery occlusion.

a) Occlusion of the Central Retinal Vein

Ophthalmoscopic Finding (Figs. 80–82)

Disc:
Color: Red; hyperemia of the capillaris on the disc.
Form and Size: Apparently increased.
Margins: Blurred, slightly prominent, surrounded by hemorrhages.
Vessels: Arterioles attenuated, variations in caliber: The veins are markedly
                      dilated, tortuous and dark. Arteriovenous crossing phenomena;
                      some of the vessels are covered by blood, later by neovasculariza-
                      tion (rete mirabilis formation, Fig. 82).
Retina: Numerous flame-shaped hemorrhages reaching into the periphery;
                      later: light, degenerative areas.

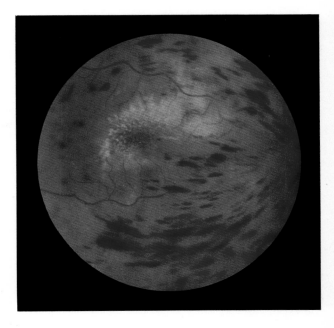

Fig. 81. Occlusion of the central retinal vein (thrombosis); hemorrhages and degenerative foci also in the macular area.

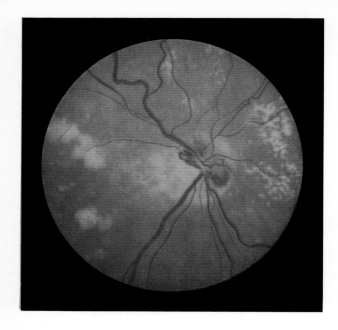

Fig. 82. Old occlusion (thrombosis) of the central retinal vein. On the disc numerous newly formed blood vessels (so-called rete mirabilis). The veins are still somewhat dilated. Numerous degenerative foci all over the fundus.

b) Occlusion of a Branch of the Central Retinal Vein

Ophthalmoscopic Finding (Figs. 83, 84)

If only one or two branches of the central vein are occluded, the above described pathologic changes (hemostasis, flame-shaped hemorrhages, light degenerative areas) are found only in the retinal sector which is drained by the affected vein. Such branch occlusions originate frequently from arteriovenous crossing areas. In these areas, artery and vein have a common periadventitia. The symptoms are here less pronounced than when the central retinal vein is occluded. The patient may only complain about a "veil" over his vision. Central acuity may be unaffected.

Complications

Secondary ("neovascular") glaucoma, ascending (retinal) optic atrophy.

Differential Diagnosis

Papilledema (page 70).

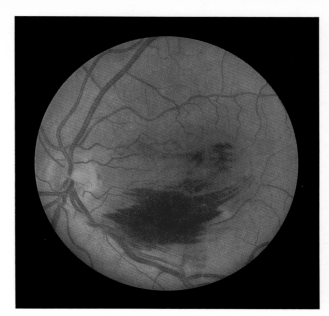

Fig. 83. Occlusion of a branch of the central retinal vein (thrombosis). The lower temporal segment is affected. In the area supplied by the inferior temporal vein are extensive hemorrhages reaching into the macula.

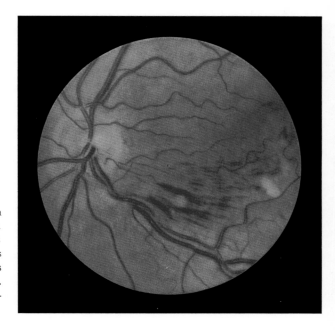

Fig. 84. Occlusion of a branch of the central retinal vein (thrombosis). Same case as Fig. 83, but after two weeks of treatment; the hemorrhages are more or less absorbed. There are a few, light degenerative foci.

5. Periphlebitis (Juvenile, Recurrent Vitreous Hemorrhages)

General

The retinal periphlebitis (Eales's disease) is an insidious inflammation of the walls of the retinal veins. This leads to hemorrhages into the vitreous with sudden loss of vision and without premonitory symptoms. The hemorrhages appear as a black wall or as a brown-red moving curtain. The vitreous may be filled with blood and only after absorption of the blood can the fundus be seen. The disease is characterized by many recurrences which may vary in intensity and in duration. The disease occurs more frequently in males than in females. The patients are otherwise completely normal. The disease is also called "juvenile, recurrent retinal and vitreous hemorrhages." The first hemorrhages usually lie in the periphery. Blood from even extensive and nearly blinding hemorrhages may eventually be absorbed. The prognosis is better in young patients than in older ones. We distinguish an exudative, a hemorrhagic, and a proliferative type. In severe cases with poor absorption of the blood, irreversible scars will form. Blindness is then due to dense vitreous opacities, preretinal membranes, and a proliferation of connective tissue and vessels (retinitis proliferans, Fig. 88) and secondary retinal detachment (page 140).

The etiology of this disease is not known. It is possible that hormonal factors or toxic-allergic reactions play a role. Occasionally one finds increased erythro-poiesis in the bone marrow and an increased number of erythrocytes in the peripheral blood.

Ophthalmoscopic Finding (Figs. 85–88)

Disc: Normal color, sharply outlined.

Vessels: Arteries: Normal; arteriovenous anastomosis (neovascularization) (Fig. 87).

Veins: In *acute* cases there are fluffy, yellow-white infiltrates (Fig. 85); in *older* cases there is a greyish-white sheathing and neovascularization close to the veins (Fig. 86).

Retina: Hemorrhages from dilated, newly formed vessels (Fig. 87).

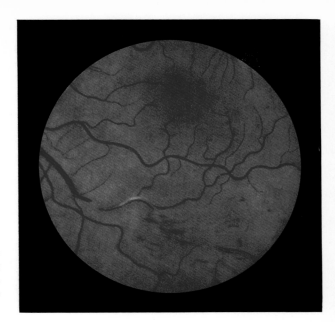

Fig. 85. Acute retinal periphlebitis. Circumscribed sheathing of the inferior temporal veins. A few flame-shaped hemorrhages.

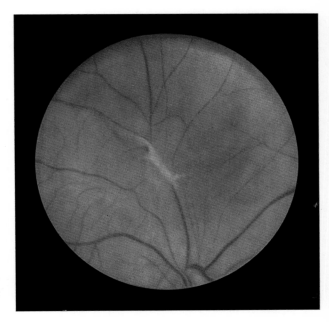

Fig. 86. Old retinal periphlebitis: Sheathing of the superior temporal vein.

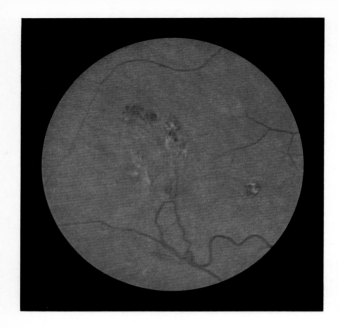

Fig. 87. Retinal periphlebitis. Numerous newly formed blood vessels in addition to hemorrhages and degenerative foci.

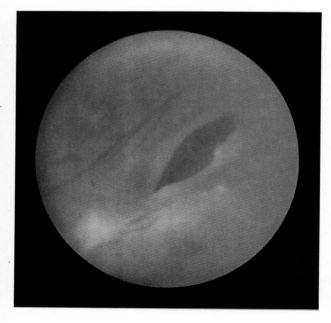

Fig. 88. Proliferative retinopathy after periphlebitis with formation of a tear in the retina.

6. Affections of the Retina in Systemic Diseases

General

The examination of the ocular fundus is of utmost importance in numerous systemic diseases, e.g. arteriosclerosis, hypertension, diabetes, etc. The ophthalmoscopic examination may here give important diagnostic, prognostic and therapeutic clues.

We have, however, to keep in mind that the retinal vessels and the retinal tissue can, because of their anatomical structure, react to various disturbances only in very few and often uniform ways. The type and extent of the retinal changes are also conditioned by the age of the patient and the duration and course of the systemic disease.

a) Arteriosclerosis

The ophthalmoscopic signs of arteriosclerotic changes are especially manifold. This is due to the anatomic and functional peculiarities of the retinal vascular system. These changes are not only pathologic alterations of the blood vessels, which are especially well-visible on the fluorescein angiogram (Fig. 89), but also damage the resulting tissue. The former change is called "arteriosclerotic fundus," the other one "arteriosclerotic retinopathy."

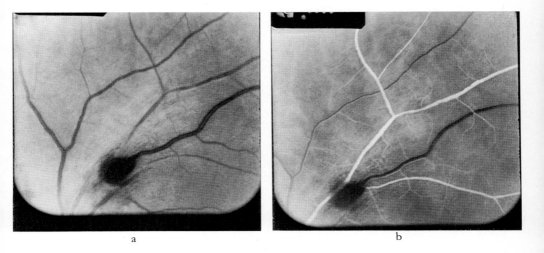

a　　　　　　　　　　　　　　　b

Fig. 89. Fluorescein angiogram of an arteriosclerotic fundus. a) Preliminary picture (with filters) before injection of the dye. b) Arterial phase. The variations in the caliber of the vessels are better visible when the vessel is filled with fluorescein. The dark areas represent hemorrhages.

Ophthalmoscopic Finding

α) Simple Arteriosclerotic Fundus (Fig. 90)

Of main importance here are changes of the retinal vessels:

Disc: Normal.

Arteries: Thickening of the vascular wall; widened, white sheathing reaching into the periphery, variations in caliber, occasionally complete occlusions.

Veins: Moderate tortuosity, especially of the venules, varicosities, crossing phenomena of Gunn (page 108).

Retina: The fundus is pale and reflexes are rare. There are occasional hemorrhages, irregularities of pigmentation, and fine degenerative foci (dyshoric foci).

If the vascular changes go beyond the vascular tree and if there is an involvement of the retina and the choroid, we speak of:

β) Arteriosclerotic Retinopathy (Figs. 91, 92)

Here we distinguish according to the fact whether the capillary permeability is decreased or increased: a dry or a wet (exudative) form.

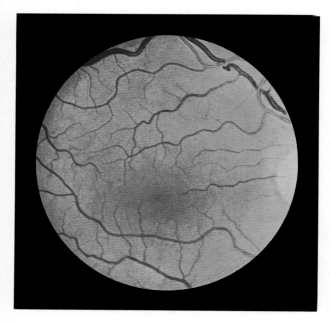

Fig. 90. Simple arteriosclerotic fundus. The fundus is pale with few reflexes. The arteries have a widened reflex and the venules are tortuous. Gunn's crossing phenomena are present.

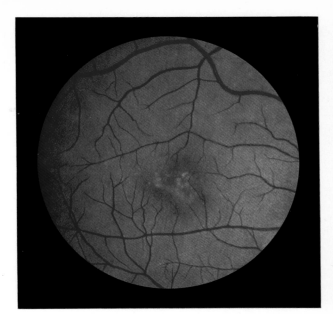

Fig. 91. Arteriosclerotic retinopathy (dry form). Pigmentary disturbances at the posterior pole, numerous dyshoric foci.

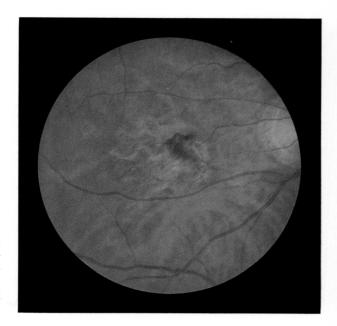

Fig. 92. Arteriosclerotic retinopathy (wet form). Hemorrhages at the posterior pole (disciform macula degeneration). In addition there is choroidal sclerosis.

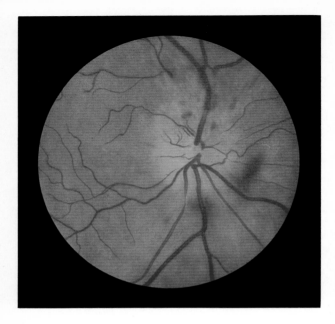

Fig. 93. Ischemic neuropathy. The disc is pale and shows blurred outlines. Peripapillary hemorrhages, attenuated arteries with irregular caliber.

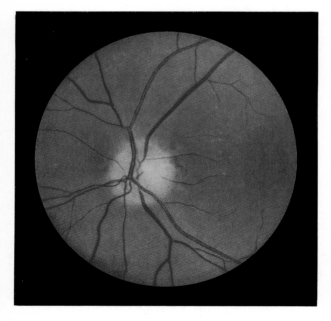

Fig. 94. Ischemic optic atrophy. The disc is pale and slightly blurred. The arteries show sclerotic changes.

1. *The Dry Form:* (Fig. 91)

Disc: Normal color and sharply outlined.

Vessels: See arteriosclerotic fundus (page 104).

Retina: Degenerative foci, partly white, partly pigmented in the macular
       area (Fig. 91) and in the retinal periphery; in case of obliteration
       of retinal vessels a cystoid degeneration may develop in the retinal
       periphery mainly due to the chronically poor vascularization
       (Fig. 121). Development of retinal tears with retinal detachment
       (page 135).

2. *The Wet Form:* (Fig. 92) Retinal hemorrhages with disciform degeneration of the
retina (KUHNT-JUNIUS) (page 132).

The pathologic changes found in choroidal sclerosis are described on page 161.

Complications

Occlusion of the central retinal artery (page 92).
Occlusion of the central retinal vein (page 96).
Vascular pseudopapillitis (page 70).

This type of arteriosclerotic disease of the optic nerve is also called *"ischemic neuropathy"* or *"vascular pseudopapillitis."* It occurs in elderly patients with systemic arteriosclerosis. The ophthalmoscopic picture differs from that of an inflammatory neuritis or papillitis (page 67) by the early pallor of the blurred disc, flame-shaped hemorrhages and a diffuse sclerosis of the retinal arterioles. Because of the sclerosis of the nutrient vessels of the optic nerve an ischemic infarct with necrosis may be found microscopically (KREIBIG). Clinically, the end-result will be a vascular optic atrophy (Fig. 94).

γ) The Relationship Between Ocular Fundus Changes and Systemic Disease

Patients with an arteriosclerotic fundus frequently have pathologic findings in the serum (hypercholesterolemia, increase in serum fat, increase in neutral glyco-proteins, diminished serum proteins). But these variations are not always present, similar to their inconsistent behavior in other forms of arteriosclerosis (sclerosis of the coronary, cerebral and peripheral vessels). Arteriosclerosis of the retinal vessels is often combined with similar changes in other vascular systems.

b) Hypertension

General

The ophthalmoscopic picture differs according to the type of hypertension. It is different in cases of benign, red (stages 1 and 2) and malignant, renal, pale (stages 2 and 3) hypertension.

There are many cases which fall between these two types, and hypertension may frequently be accompanied by arteriosclerosis (page 103). In any case the ophthalmoscopic picture may give the internist clues as to the necessity of further diagnostic examinations and to the prognosis of the diseases.

α) Hypertonic Retinopathy

(Ocular Fundus in the so-called Benign, Red or Essential Hypertension)

Ophthalmoscopic Finding (Figs. 95–99)

(Usually bilateral)

Disc:	Sharply outlined and normal in color.
Arterioles:	Well-filled, broad, golden-yellow reflex (copper-wire arteries), tortuous and of irregular caliber.
Veins:	The larger ones are filled and dilated. The venules around the macular area are markedly tortuous (Guist sign). At the arterio-venous crossing the vein may show an arcuate deviation (Salus sign) or the vein appears interrupted in the area where it is crossed by the arteriole (Gunn sign) (Fig. 97).
	(More recent examinations [SEITZ] have shown that these changes are not due to a true compression of the vein, but are caused by thickening of the perivascular tissue sheath which is here common to artery and vein. Originally, these crossing phenomena were thought to be pathognomic for hypertension. Presently we no longer think so. Similar changes have been observed in arteriosclerosis without hypertension. In addition, there is no relation between the degree and the number of the crossing phenomena and the severity of the hypertensive cardiovascular disease.)
Retina:	The entire fundus appears deep red (Fig. 95) with numerous reflexes and a few small hemorrhages. There are very small, white-yellow degenerative foci, greyish areas of edema as an expression of disturbed vascular permeability (Figs. 97–99).

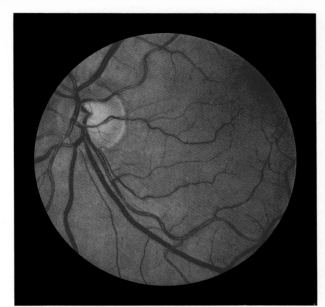

Fig. 95. Hypertonic retinopathy. The disc is sharply outlined and the fundus deep red. The arterioles are tortuous and filled with a golden-yellow reflex. The venules are markedly tortuous.

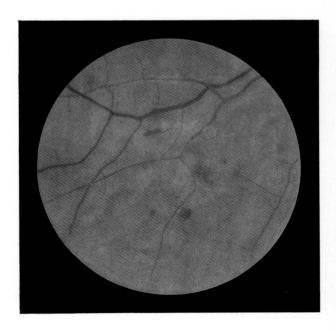

Fig. 96. Hypertonic retinopathy.

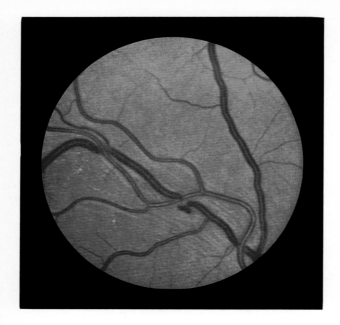

Fig. 97. Fundus in hypertension. Copper-wire arteries. The veins are dilated and there are Gunn's crossing phenomena with degenerative foci.

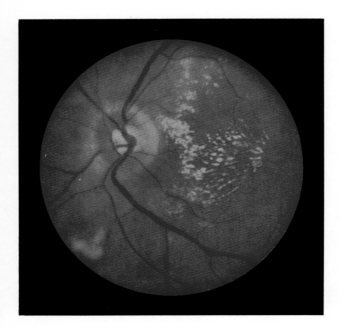

Fig. 98. Hypertensive fundus: Numerous light degenerative foci between disc and macula.

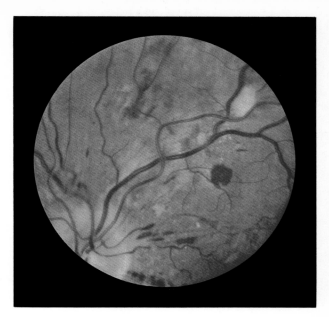

Fig. 99. Fundus in hypertension. Intermediate stage to angiospastic retinopathy. The disc margins are blurred. The arteries are attenuated and there are numerous hemorrhages.

The differentiation between a *hypertonic fundus* and a *hypertensive (angiospastic) retinopathy* with the division into various stages is primarily of *prognostic* importance. The experienced examiner can, on the basis of the findings in the ocular fundus, make as valuable predictions for the course of the disease as he can on the basis of the blood pressure values.

If we assume that the disease takes a similar course in other vascular areas, we may deduce that the presence of pathologic changes of the *retinal vessels alone* will signify that the *parenchyma* of kidney or brain, for instance, is essentially unchanged as is that of the retina. The prognosis of stage I or II of the hypertonic fundus is much better than an angiospastic retinopathy of stage I or II.

The special value of an examination of the ocular fundus in patients with hypertension lies in the fact that it enables the examiner to differentiate between the benign and the malignant variety of the disease at a time at which it is very difficult for the internist to do this. In addition, the experienced examiner may on the basis of the ophthalmoscopic findings give quite accurate predictions as to the *further course* of the disease and on the effect which therapeutic measures might have. Fundus photography will be of great value. It enables the examiner to make an exact comparison of numerous details over a long period of time. It is more accurate than a description or reliance on memory.

β) Hypertensive (Angiospastic) Retinopathy

(Ocular Fundus in Malignant, Nephrogenic, Pale Hypertension)

General

Hypertensive retinopathy is a term used for the severe pathologic changes of the ocular fundus found in patients with severe damage to the kidneys (glomerulonephritis, pyelonephritis, amyloid degeneration, diabetic nephrosis (KIMMELSTIEL-WILSON), malignant nephrosclerosis, nephropathy of pregnancy).

Previously when proteinuria was thought to be the most important sign, this condition was referred to as "albuminuric retinitis." This was at a time when it was not appreciated that the fundus changes occur when there is a disturbance of the *renal blood supply*.

The hallmark of this condition is the attenuation of the retinal arterioles. Because of reduced retinal vascularization the entire fundus appears pale (ischemic retinitis of Volhard).

Papilledema is only rarely absent. It is an expression of local permeability disturbances in the optic nerve or in the retina, or it may be the result of an increase in intra-cranial pressure.

Ophthalmoscopic Finding (Figs. 100, 101)

(Usually Bilateral)

Disc:	Hyperemic because of venous stasis, blurred margins, slight elevation, diameter apparently increased, vessels elevated in the edematous area, hemorrhages close to the vessels.
Arterioles:	Extremely attenuated especially in the area close to the disc, glistening, light reflex stripes and sheathing (silver-wire arteries); partly transformed into white cords, variations in caliber, small arterioles extremely thin, hardly visible.
Veins:	Initially unchanged, later stasis, relation of arteriolar to venous caliber 1:3, Salus sign present, numerous conspicuous Gunn phenomena.
Retina:	The fundus is pale, flame-shaped hemorrhages, also peripherally close to the arterioles; circumpapillary ischemic edema; numerous white, fluffy, cotton-wool exudates, degenerative foci often in groups or in the form of a macular star (Figs. 100, 101).

On the basis of the ophthalmoscopic picture we can say that the *prognosis* is poor when there is pronounced edema, hemorrhages and a macular star. These are signs of a vascular damage due to toxins and hypertension.

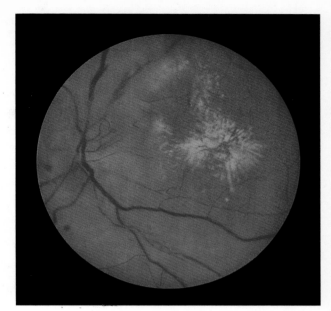

Fig. 100. Hypertensive retinopathy: The fundus is pale, papilledema, arterioles markedly attenuated, the small branches hardly visible, a few hemorrhages nasally and below. Degenerative foci in the macular area forming a "macular star."

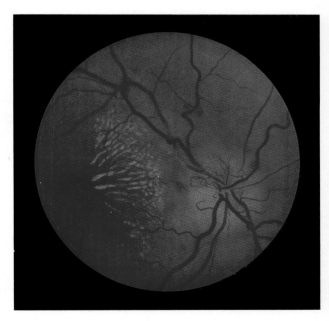

Fig. 101. Hypertensive retinopathy (see above).

c) Nephropathy of Pregnancy

If the changes of an angiospastic retinopathy occur in a pregnant woman, we speak of a *retinopathy of pregnancy*.

This occurs during the last trimester of pregnancy with hypertension, albuminuria, *spasm* of the retinal arterioles with hemorrhages and marked exudative changes in the retina (serous detachment) and disc (papilledema). These findings indicate a severe toxic status. These pathologic changes are, *at least initially*, not caused by any *organic* vascular disturbance and the condition may, therefore, regress completely after delivery, provided there is no chronic damage to the kidneys. Regular and careful ophthalmoscopic control is necessary.

Ophthalmoscopic Finding (Fig. 102)

See hypertensive retinopathy in malignant, pale hypertension (page 112).

Occasionally we many encounter in *eclampsia* a type of blindness which is of central origin. In these patients the ocular fundus is normal. We must assume that this is due to a disturbance of vascular supply to the visual cortex.

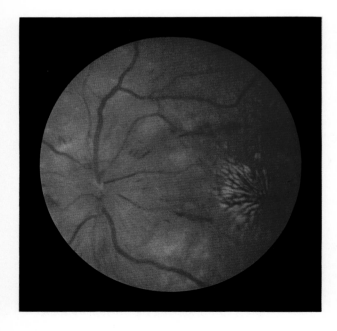

Fig. 102. Retinopathy of pregnancy. Edema of the disc and the retina. The arterioles are spastically attenuated. There are flame-shaped hemorrhages and a group of degenerative foci in the macula.

Differential Diagnosis

	Arteriosclerosis	Hypertonic Retinopathy	Hypertensive Retinopathy
Papilledema	(+)	—	+
Arterioles:			
Tortuosity	—	++	+
Caliber	Attenuated	Dilated	Markedly attenuated
Variations in Caliber	+	+	++
Reflex Stripes	+	+	++
		Copper-wire arteries	Silver-wire arteries
Gunn Sign	+	+	+++
Salus Sign	(+)	+	+++
Guist Sign	—	+	—
Retina:			
Hemorrhages	+	(+)	++
Cotton-wool Spots	—	—	++
Fatty Degenerations	+	+	+
Edema	—	—	+
Macular Star	—	(+)	+

d) Diseases Due to the Occlusion of Large Arteries

In addition to the above mentioned vascular diseases ocular symptoms occur also in obliterative processes of the carotid and the subclavian arteries. In these cases the blood supply to the brain is interfered with.

α) Occlusion of the Internal Carotid

An occlusion of the internal carotid, which was first described by VIRCHOW in 1856 as a thrombosis, occurs in older patients and is usually due to arteriosclerosis. In 75% of the cases the occlusion lies close to the branching from the external carotid. The clinical picture is protean because of numerous anastomoses. The patients complain about transient, frequently changing, unilateral visual disturbances and obscurations. There are hardly any prodromal symptoms and there is no pain. In more advanced cases the patient experiences blindness on the side of the occlusion and a hemiplegia on the other side. If we are dealing with an acute complete occlusion, the ophthalmoscopic examination shows an ischemia of the retina (page 92), but the occlusion is usually slowly progressive. Therefore, we find in the fundus pathologic changes corresponding to the underlying disease, which is usually a severe arteriosclerosis (page 104) and in addition there are cotton-wool patches, retinal hemorrhages, papilledema and primary optic atrophy. The diagnosis can be made with the help of x-rays, ophthalmodynamometry, and dynamography.

β) The Syndrome of the Aortic Arch

The aortic arch syndrome (Takayasu) is due to inflammatory processes (syphilis) and occlusion of the *subclavian artery*. It is frequently found in young females. There is no pulsation in the large vessels coming from the aortic arch ("Pulseless disease"). The patient experiences because of decreased blood flow unilateral, frequently right-sided visual disturbances which are more pronounced when the patient walks or works than when he is lying down. The decreased blood flow to the head and neck area may lead to a degeneration of the iris and the lens. The retinal arterioles show fragmentation of blood flow and tortuosity. The veins are dilated. There are also arteriovenous anastomoses, microaneurysms, degenerative foci, pigmentary disturbances, and atrophy of the optic nerve.

γ) Temporal Arteritis (Giant Cell Arteritis)
General

Temporal arteritis (Horton) also belongs to the diseases which may lead to vascular occlusions. It occurs in patients of advanced age and may be the cause of a very sudden visual disturbance or blindness.

The patient frequently has a slightly elevated temperature, severe headaches, markedly increased sedimentation rate of the erythrocytes. The temporal artery is often thickened, tortuous, and tender (Fig. 103a). No pulse can be palpated. The acute visual disturbance or blindness is due to an occlusion of the nutrient vessel of the optic nerve, this may lead to a unilateral (occasionally bilateral) optico-malacia (KREIBIG). The final proof for the correct diagnosis is the histologic picture (Fig. 103b) of the biopsy of an affected artery (giant cell arteritis). The prognosis as far as vision is concerned is poor.

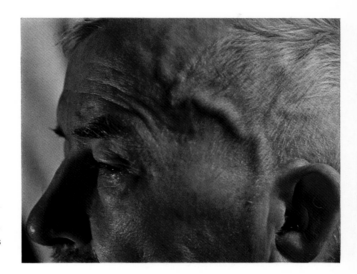

Fig. 103a. Temporal arteritis. The temporal artery is indurated and tortuous.

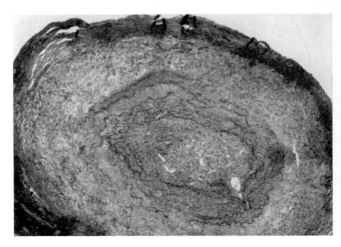

Fig. 103b. Histologic findings. Occlusion of the lumen through hyperplasia of the intima. Destruction of media and adventitia by granulomatous inflammation.

Ophthalmoscopic Finding (Fig. 104)

Disc: In acute cases, pale, slightly elevated (ischemic papilledema may cause ischemic neuritis); the margins are blurred and later the borders may be sharply outlined.

Arterioles: As in arteriosclerotic fundus (page 104).

Veins: Unchanged; Gunn and Salus signs are present.

Retina: A few hemorrhages.

Differential Diagnosis

Ischemic neuropathy due to other diseases (page 107).
Arteriosclerotic optic atrophy (page 107).

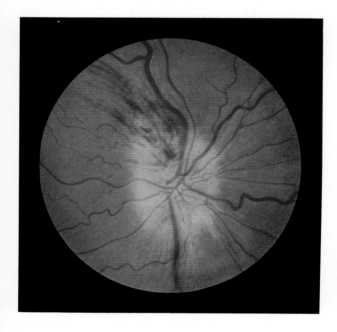

Fig. 104. Temporal arteritis. The disc is pale and shows blurred outlines. Arteriosclerosis of the vessels, retinal hemorrhages.

e) Diabetes Mellitus

General

Nearly all parts of the eye can be affected in diabetes. The diabetic changes of the ocular fundus are especially important for diagnosis and prognosis of the systemic disease. Diabetic retinopathy is becoming one of the most frequent causes of blindness. The appearance of a diabetic retinopathy (TH. LEBER, 1875) depends not only on the severity of the diabetic metabolic disorder, but also on the age of the patient when the disease first appears, on the duration of the disease, and on certain hereditary factors. When and if, during the course of the disease, a diabetic retinopathy occurs depends more or less on the regulation of the diabetes. Usually retinopathy does not occur before the disease has been present for 5 to 10 years. After 15 or more years of disease nearly 60% of the patients have a retinopathy. Young patients are relatively more often affected than old ones. Great variations of the blood sugar level, when the metabolic anomaly cannot be regulated by diet or with medications, seem to aggravate the retinopathy. The sudden appearance of microaneurysms and small retinal hemorrhages may be the first indication that the diabetes is not well controlled. Depending on the type and

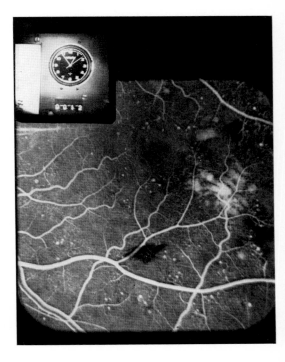

Fig. 105. Fluorescein angiogram in diabetic retinopathy. Capillary phase. After injection of fluorescein, numerous microaneurysms (visible in the picture as light dots) become apparent. The hemorrhages are dark areas. The exudates appear as large, light spots.

the extent of the retinal changes the visual acuity may suffer. Fluorescein angiography (page 17) demonstrates especially well the true changes in the retinal vessels. It shows the number and the site of the microaneurysms better than ordinary ophthalmoscopy (Fig. 105). These pathologic changes are bilateral and, in the beginning, mainly located around the disc and at the posterior pole. Later on one also finds retinal exudates which can lead to neovascularization and to recurrent vitreous hemorrhages. Finally, there may be a scar tissue transformation of large retinal areas, neovascularization on the retina, and preretinal membranes and scars (proliferative retinopathy, Fig. 109). A secondary detachment may follow (page 140). Arteriosclerotic (page 103) and hypertensive (page 108) vascular changes may occur simultaneously in middle-aged or old patients. Some authors claim that in the early stages light coagulation of the microorganisms and of the bleeding vessels may beneficially influence the course of the disease. Occasionally, even in advanced stages this type of treatment may be of benefit. Every diabetic patient should have his ocular fundi examined regularly and frequently. Other ocular complications of diabetes are rubeosis of the iris with neovascularization in the chamber angle and neovascular glaucoma, diabetic cataract, and (rarely) optic neuropathy.

Ophthalmoscopic Finding (Figs. 106–109)

(Usually bilateral)

Disc: Normal in color and sharp outlines.

Vessels: The precapillaries show fusiform dilatations, the veins are dilated, neovascularization (rete mirabilis).

Retina: Early stage (Fig. 106): Between the temporal vessels are irregular, disseminated, dot-like and flame-shaped red spots and areas (microaneurysms and hemorrhages). There are polygonal, sharply outlined foci at the posterior pole. These coalesce or are arranged in a wreath-like fashion (Figs. 106-108).

These deposits are an expression of lipid degeneration and organization of hemorrhages. Frequently, hemorrhages surround them in a typical "horseshoe-shaped" fashion.

Late stage (Fig. 109): Rete mirabilis formation of the blood vessels, preretinal strands and scars (proliferative retinopathy), eventually secondary retinal detachment.

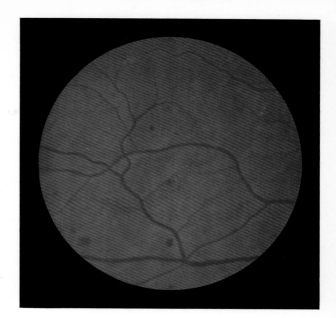

Fig. 106. Diabetic retinopathy (early stage). A few dot-like hemorrhages at the posterior pole and small, light degenerative foci.

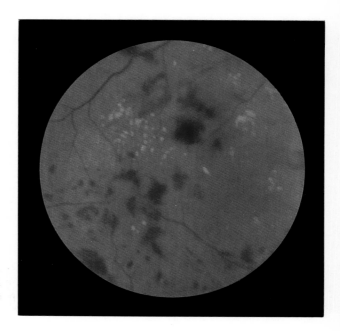

Fig. 107. Diabetic retinopathy. Numerous hemorrhages and degenerative deposits at the posterior pole.

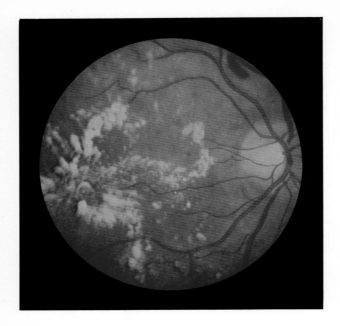

Fig. 108. Diabetic retinopathy. Numerous polygonal, sharply outlined, degenerative foci. They are partly coalescing, and partly in a wreath-like arrangement.

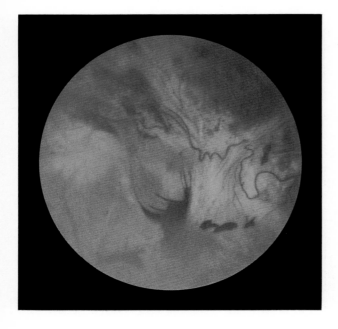

Fig. 109. Proliferative retinopathy in diabetes. Hemorrhages, neovascularization, and pre-retinal bands.

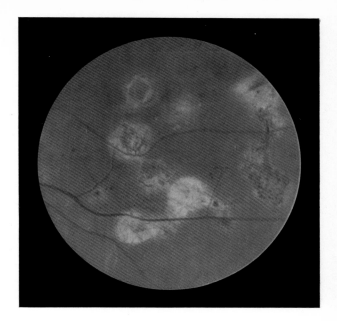

Fig. 110. Diabetic retinopathy. The microaneurysms were lightcoagulated. Hemorrhages and beginning scarring.

α) Diabetic Nephrosclerosis (Kimmelstiel-Wilson)

General

Hypertension and arteriosclerosis occur especially early in juvenile diabetics and are more frequently seen in males than in females. Over the course of years the primary disease may cause a renal decompensation and a diabetic nephropathy (intercapillary glomerulosclerosis) with albuminuria edema and uremia. In addition to the above described diabetic retinal changes these patients also show papilledema and retinal edema, cotton-wool spots, and ischemic areas. These findings are not pathognomonic for Kimmelstiel-Wilson disease, but may also occur in other severe affections of the kidneys due to causes other than diabetes.

Ophthalmoscopic Finding

Disc: Edematous, blurred outlines.
Arteries: The arterioles may be unchanged or markedly attenuated. There
            are greyish-white sheathings along the vessels. Small arterioles
            are hardly visible. Rows of microaneurysms.
Veins: Tortuous.
Retina: Dot-like and flame-shaped hemorrhages, cotton-wool patches,
            degenerative deposits frequently as macular star.

f) Diseases of the Blood and the Hematopoietic Organs

Typical changes in the ocular fundus can be seen in various diseases of the blood and the hematopoietic organs causing disturbances of leuko- or erythropoiesis, or changes in the peripheral blood.

α) Anemia

General

An "anemic retinopathy" can be seen accompanying any case of severe anemia. A marked pallor of the fundus – as seen in the mucous membranes – is the most conspicuous change. In this way we get a fundus picture similar to that seen in occlusion of the central retinal artery (page 92).

Ophthalmoscopic Finding

Disc: Edematous, blurred outlines.
Vessels: Arterioles and veins narrow, nearly bloodless. Partly obscured by retinal edema.
Retina: Opaque, edematous, yellowish deposits with surrounding hemorrhages.

β) Polycythemia

General

A dark-red discoloration of the fundus with marked tortuosity of the veins (retinal cyanosis) occurs with increase in the number of red blood cells (polycythemia). This corresponds to the cyanosis of the face and of the mucous membranes.

Ophthalmoscopic Finding

Disc: Occasionally edematous and elevated (papilledema).
Vessels: Arterioles slightly dilated; veins dilated, appear nearly black.
Retina: Dot-like hemorrhages; small greyish-white foci; the entire fundus appears dark-red to bluish.

Similar changes in the ocular fundus with retinal hemorrhages, edema, degenerative and proliferative changes, and occasionally with optic atrophy may also be seen in:

>Thrombopenia,
>Hemophilia and
>Hodgkin's Disease.

γ) Leukemia

General

The pale yellow discoloration of the fundus (leukemic retinopathy) is typical for this disease. In addition, we frequently find retinal hemorrhages, degenerative

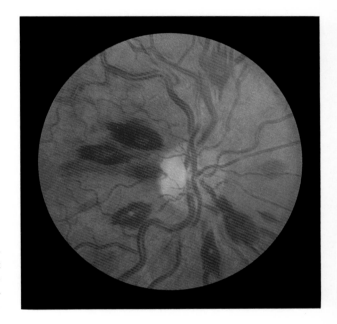

Fig. 111. Leukemic retinopathy. The fundus is light yellow. The veins are tortuous, dilated and there are numerous retinal hemorrhages.

deposits and alterations of the blood vessels. These changes will not allow a classification of the leukemia present. Occasionally, the enormous number of leukocytes will give the vessels a nearly milky appearance. Sometimes a true papilledema is present. The cause for this may be the increased blood viscosity, the increased capillary permeability, leukemic infiltrates in the optic nerve, or an increase in the intracranial pressure.

Ophthalmoscopic Finding

Disc:	Blurred margins, edematous; occasionally elevated (papilledema).
Vessels:	The arterioles rarely are of a milky color; the veins are dilated and tortuous.
Retina:	Light yellow to greyish deposits and infiltrates (leukemic infiltrates). These are frequently surrounded by a hemorrhage.

δ) Macroglobulinemia (Waldenström)

General

Numerous pathologic conditions may lead to pathologic alteration of the serum proteins. If there is a quantitative disturbance, we speak of *dysproteinemia*. If foreign proteins appear, we call it *paraproteinemia.*

In macroglobulinemia we usually find heavy paraproteins in the serum which because of their high molecular weight (approximately 1,000,000) are called macroglobulins. Electrophoretic examination and ultracentrifugal differentiation will separate these proteins from the normal serum proteins. These pathologic proteins cause an increase in the viscosity of the blood and disturbances of vascular permeability and of blood coagulation A markedly increased sedimentation rate and a tendency for bleeding are the most prominent clinical signs.

The "sludged blood" phenomenon with fragmentation of the blood column and slowing of the blood current can be seen in the conjunctival vessels. This phenomenon corresponds to the increase in sedimentation rate.

Changes in the blood viscosity and the presence of paraproteins may produce a fundus picture sometimes referred to as *"visco-paraproteinemic fundus."* It is primarily characterized by alterations of the venous system.

Ophthalmoscopic Finding

(Nearly always bilateral)

Disc:	Edematous, blurred margins.
Arterioles:	Unchanged.
Veins:	Tortuous, dilated, varicosities and constrictions (sausage-like appearance). With pressure on the globe there is fragmentation of the blood column.
Retina:	Numerous perivenous hemorrhages reaching into the periphery, exudative foci, edema, serous retinal detachment (page 140).

Differential Diagnosis

Papilledema (page 70).
Occlusion of the Central Retinal Vein (page 96) but this is rarely bilateral.

g) Septicemia

General

Hematogenous dissemination of infectious material into the retinal capillaries may occur in septicemia. This may lead to an increase in the permeability of the vascular walls or to a uni- or bilateral true retinitis (septic retinitis of Roth). Complete restitution of sight depends upon the course of the disease.

Ophthalmoscopic Finding

Disc: Normal.
Vessels: Unchanged.
Retina: Small, grey, fluffy retinal foci lie close to the vessels (Roth spots); small dot-like hemorrhages.

If the number and virulence of the infectious organism are high and if the resistance of the host is low, the intraocular inflammation may be much more extensive and lead to the so-called *metastatic ophthalmia*. This is characterized by severe pain, exophthalmos, lid edema, chemosis, ciliary injection of the globe, protein and pus in the anterior chamber and the vitreous (formation of an abscess).

7. Diseases of the Macula

General

The macula is a circumscribed topographical area which has a very definite anatomical structure and specialized function (pages 34, 46). Some disease processes occur characteristically only in the macular area. Such processes will usually produce a marked loss of function (decreased visual acuity, central scotoma, metamorphopsia). Even if such complaints point toward a macular disease, the examination of the macula should be done at the end of the ophthalmoscopic evaluation (page 46).

In order to examine the macular area the patient has to look straight ahead into the light of the ophthalmoscope (Fig. 7). Using the usual light the macula appears darker than the surrounding fundus; some details (macular and foveolar reflex, yellow pigmentation) are visible only when red-free illumination is used (page 46).

We distinguish between congenital, inflammatory, traumatic, senile, and myopic macular diseases.

a) The Congenital Macular Diseases

α) Congenital Aplasia of the Macula

Ophthalmoscopic Finding (For instance in albinism)

Disc: Normal color and sharply outlined, but difficult to distinguish from the pole surrounding.
Vessels: Normal, the choroidal vessels are visible.
Retina and Choroid: There is little pigment in the fundus, the normal yellow of the macula and the normal macular reflexes are absent.

β) Coloboma (page 49)

γ) Hereditary Degenerations (Infantile, juvenile, virile, or senile)

Ophthalmoscopic Finding

Disc: Normal color and sharply outlined.
Vessels: Normal.
Retina: Cystoid or punched-out degenerations in the area of the macula. They usually are disc-shaped, often oval, larger than the macula itself. There are disturbances of pigmentation and atrophic areas.

b) Inflammatory Diseases

The macula can be the site of an isolated, primary inflammation. This is the case in a so-called *central chorioretinitis* (page 158). Toxoplasmosis preferentially affects the macular area (Fig. 112, and page 158).

Ophthalmoscopic Finding (Fig. 112)

Disc: Normal color and sharply outlined.
Vessels: Normal.
Retina and choroid: In the macula area and surrounding a large atrophic focus
               with pigmentation in the center and at the margin.

Often the macular area is *secondarily* affected in the course of a proliferating inflammation, for instance a *retinal periphlebitis* (page 100).

The macula may also show changes when other parts of the eye are inflamed. A diffuse *choroiditis* or a chronic *iridocyclitis* may lead to an edema or to a cystoid degeneration of the macula.

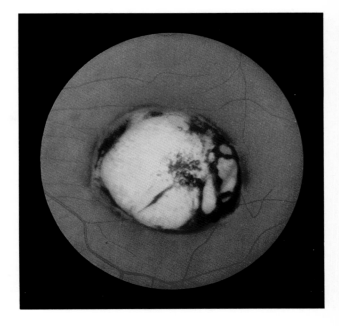

Fig. 112. Central chorioretinal scar in congenital toxoplasmosis.

c) Traumatic Macular Disease

It is seen more frequently after a blunt than after a perforating injury.

α) Berlin's Edema (page 150)

(Vascular damage by a "Contre-Coup" effect on the retina)

Ophthalmoscopic Finding (Fig. 131)

Disc: Normal color and fluffy outlines.
Arterioles: Attenuated (temporarily).
Retina: Circumscribed, greyish-white opacification and edema on the temporal side. The macula appears as a red spot; occasionally retinal or preretinal hemorrhages, later star-like folds in the adjacent retina sometimes leading to slight pigmentation.

β) Central Choroiditis (Retinitis Solaris)

This is due to burning with infrared light, for instance after observing an eclipse with an unprotected eye. The damage depends upon the duration and intensity of the injury. A central scotoma will result because of scar formation in the macula.

Ophthalmoscopic Finding (Fig. 113)

Disc: Normal and sharply outlined.
Retina: The normal macular reflex is absent, circumscribed edema of the central retina.
Choroid: Later on pigmentary disturbances and scar formation.

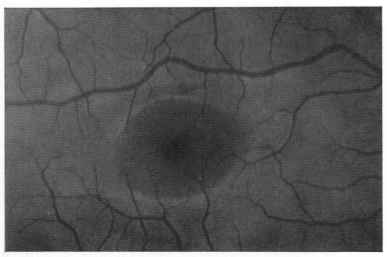

Fig. 113. Traumatic macular damage (retinitis solaris) after watching an eclipse.

γ) Formation of a Hole or Radial Hemorrhages

(After contusions caused by severe force)

Ophthalmoscopic Finding (Fig. 114)

Disc: Normal color and sharply outlined.
Retina: The macula is extremely thin or a retinal hole is present. The depth of the hole is dark red since the choroid lies bare. The margins of the hole are sharply outlined, occasionally turned over. The adjacent retina is wavy.

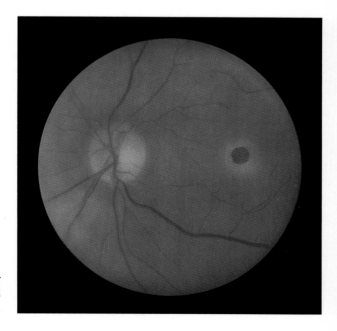

Fig. 114. Traumatic macular hole. The hole is surrounded by a narrow, edematous area.

d) Senile Changes

The macular area does not have its own arteries. It is supplied by diffusion only. It is, therefore, exquisitely vulnerable to circulatory disturbances. A sclerosis of the choriocapillaries is frequently the cause for such pathologic changes which in the end-stage may result in a disciform degeneration of the macula (Kuhnt-Junius degeneration).

Ophthalmoscopic Finding (Figs. 115, 116)

Disc: Normal color and sharply outlined.

Vessels: Arteriosclerosis (page 104).

Retina and Choroid: Greyish-white, disc-shaped opacity at the posterior pole, sub- and intraretinal exudation later, surrounded by hemorrhages, slight elevation, followed by connective tissue proliferation with uneven surface *(senile pseudotumor)* around it there may be a wreath of fatty-like deposits (circinate retinopathy) and pigmentation.

Differential Diagnosis

Choroidal Melanoma (page 164).

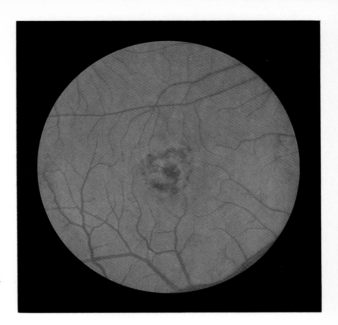

Fig. 115. Senile macular degeneration. Irregularities of pigmentation and fine scars at the posterior pole of the fundus.

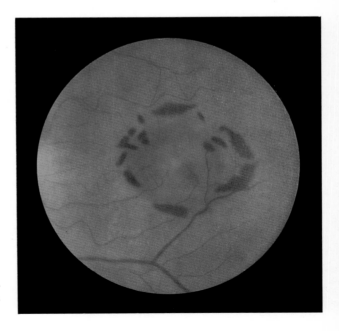

Fig. 116. Senile disciform macular degeneration (KUHNT-JUNIUS, see above).

e) Myopic Degenerations

In axial myopia the sagittal diameter of the eye is enlarged (page 23). This may produce an exophthalmos-like picture. It may lead to stretch effects on the choroid and the retina, especially at the posterior pole. In minimal myopia we usually find only a temporal choroidal atrophy (myopic conus, Fig. 50). In severe myopia we find, in addition to a peripapillary choroidal atrophy (Fig. 51), extensive degenerative areas at the posterior pole and, therefore, also in the macula. Initially, only pigmentary disturbances appear; later on degenerative areas develop with lacquer cracks and finally a greyish-black spot (Fuchs spot) appears in the foveal area which increases in size, is often surrounded by hemorrhages, and causes visual disturbances.

Ophthalmoscopic Finding (Fig. 117)

Disc: Normal color and sharply outlined.
Vessels: Straight.
Retina and Choroid: Pericapillary choroidal atrophy: The eyeground is light; round or oval atrophic areas of varying size. In these areas the sclera is visible. Pigmentary disturbances and hemorrhages in the center (Fuchs spot).

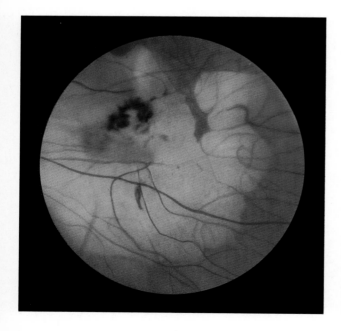

Fig. 117. Macular damage in high myopia: Large geographic atrophic areas of choroid and retina. The light sclera shines through. Pigmentation in the center (Fuchs spot).

8. Degenerative Diseases of the Retina

a) Retinitis Pigmentosa

Retinitis pigmentosa belongs to the so-called tapetoretinal degenerations. These are hereditary, degenerative diseases of the retina or the choriocapillaris. They progress during life. The *typical pigmentosa* is often of the recessive hereditary type and affects males more often than females. It is practically always a bilateral disease. In the histologic picture inflammatory changes are absent. It is a primary, progressive abiotrophy of the external retinal layers. This is accompanied by proliferation of the retinal pigment epithelium and sclerosis of the retinal vessels. Initially, already in adolescence, only the *middle zone* of the fundus is affected. Correspondingly, the patients experience first a visual disturbance of the retinal *periphery* with night blindness and a *ring scotoma* of the visual field. In the course of the disease the visual field constricts.

In the late stages the entire fundus shows pathologic changes. In the far periphery are fine pigmented granules similar to a salt and pepper fundus. The patients are practically blind because of the tunnel-like constriction of the visual field (Fig. 118). Only a small central field remains, which may leave good central visual acuity for some time. The electroretinogram, which is the electric response of the deep retinal layers to light stimulus, is usually extinguished. This degenerative disease is sometimes associated with systemic degenerative anomalies such as polydactyly and adipositas (Laurence-Moon-Biedl) and numerous other degenerative changes.

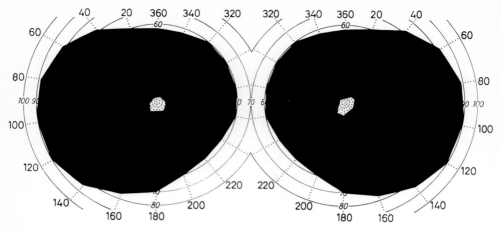

Fig. 118. Tubular visual field in retinitis pigmentosa.

Ophthalmoscopic Finding (Figs. 119, 120)

Disc:
Waxy color, pale yellow (retinal yellow atrophy, page 81) (ascending optic atrophy because of progressive degeneration of the external retinal layers, later including the retinal ganglion cells). The margins are somewhat blurred.

Vessels:
The arterioles are markedly attenuated (thread-like), often sclerotic with white sheathing. In the periphery they may be completely occluded or partly obscured by the pigment. The veins are less affected, but are also attenuated. The sclerotic choroidal vessels are visible because of atrophy of the pigment epithelium.

Retina:
Fine, branching, and star-like retinal pigmentation *(bone-corpuscle shape)*. These brown-black dots lie first in the intermediate zone and the periphery of the eyeground. The pigmentations are often connected with each other showing fine extensions. This gives the fundus a net-like appearance. The macular area remains free for a long period of time, but later on there is often a cystoid macular degeneration.

Differential Diagnosis

Disseminated Chorioretinitis (page 153).
Syphilitic Chorioretinitis (page 160).

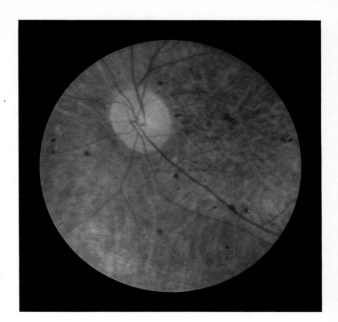

Fig. 119. Retinitis pigmentosa with retinal (waxy-yellow) optic atrophy. The blood vessels are thin. There are few bone-corpuscle-like pigmentations.

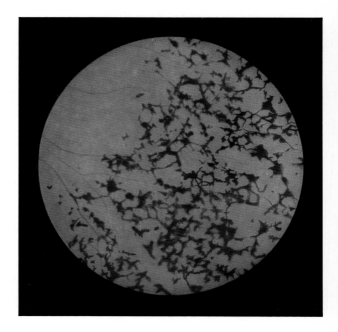

Fig. 120. Retinitis pigmentosa. Bone-corpuscle-like pigmentation of the equatorial and peripheral retina.

b) Atypical Pigmentary Degenerations of the Retina

The atypical forms differ from the typical retinitis pigmentosa insofar as the pigmentation here is only sparsely present or totally absent.

α) Retinitis Pigmentosa Sine Pigmento

With the exception of the pigmentation the changes of the disc (waxy-yellow atrophy) and of the vessels (thread-like) are identical to those of retinitis pigmentosa (see above). It can be regarded as an early stage of the same disease. The fundi are often dark and lusterless.

β) Retinitis Punctata Albescens

In this condition we find numerous, diffusely distributed, small, glistening, retinal foci. They occupy the entire eyeground. Disc and vessels may be normal or may show changes similar to those found in retinitis pigmentosa (see above). This is also a hereditary disease. It may alternate with retinitis pigmentosa in one family and the two conditions are, therefore, probably genetically related. This disease has to be differentiated from the stationary fundus albipunctatus with hemeralopia, which has normal vessels and disc.

γ) Progressive Essential Choroidal Atrophy

Progressive essential choroidal atrophy occurs as an intermediate sex-linked disease mainly only in men and in the course of time develops into almost complete choroid atrophy (Fig.144).

δ) Tapetoretinal Degenerations with Inborn Metabolic Errors

In this group of diseases cerebral lesions are frequently combined with visual defects. Three autosomal recessive lipidoses belong to this group:

1) Tay-Sachs disease with the deposition of glycolipids in the retina and in the central nervous system.
2) Niemann-Pick disease with the deposition of phospholipids in the retina and the central nervous system.
3) Gauscher's disease with the deposition of cerebrosides in the retina and the central nervous system.

In these familial amaurotic idiocies the degeneration of the ganglion cells and the progressive ascending optic atrophy lead to blindness. In addition, there are dementia, disturbances of speech, and seizures. According to the age at onset we distinguish an infantile form (Tay-Sachs) which begins early in infancy, usually between the third and sixth months of life, and a juvenile form (Vogt-Stock-Spielmeyer), which begins between the fourth and fifth years of life. For both forms the prognosis is poor.

Ophthalmoscopic Finding
(Bilateral)

Disc: Pale yellow (retinal atrophy, page 81).

Retina: *Infantile form (Tay-Sachs):* Cherry-red spot in the macula. This is surrounded by greyish-white, opaque, retinal tissue. The normal macular reflexes are absent. There is a fine cystoid degeneration with dot-like pigmentation. The vessels are attenuated.
Juvenile form (Vogt-Stock-Spielmeyer): The macular area is dark, grey-brown. The reflexes are absent in this area. There are numerous pigmentary disturbances and atrophic areas, also in the periphery (as in the so-called "salt and pepper fundus") (page 160). The vessels are also attenuated in the periphery.

Choroid: Fine depigmentation.

Differential Diagnosis

Chorioretinitis (page 153).
Central Chorioretinitis (page 153).

ε) Angioid Streaks

The angioid streaks occur frequently as a consequence of a familial progressive disturbance of the elastic tissue. This leads to breaks in Bruch's membrane. At the same time there usually are characteristic skin changes (loss of elasticity, fine yellowish areas, light stripes and coarse folds: Pseudoxanthoma elasticum). These skin changes are often found on the neck and over the large joints (Grönblad-Strandberg syndrome).

Ophthalmoscopic Finding

Disc: Normal color and sharp outlines.

Vessels: Unchanged.

Retina: Brown-red, finely granulated lines lie under the retina. They resemble tortuous and bizarre vessels. They often course radially from the disc toward the periphery. Slate-grey discoloration of the macular area due to subretinal exudation, pigmentation, and hemorrhages.

Choroid: Areolar atrophy.

Differential-Diagnosis

Central Chorioretinitis (page 153).

9. Retinal Detachment

General

Only at the ora serrata and at the optic nervehead is the retina adherent to the underlying structures. The development of a retinal detachment depends upon the condition of the vitreous, of the retina, and of the underlying tissues.

Tears in the retina lead to a *primary* (serous) detachment as the vitreous fluid may reach through the hole to the subretinal space thereby pushing the retina away from the pigment epithelium. Such tears frequently lie in the temporal or upper temporal segment. They may also lie in the macular area or near the ora serrata. The following factors may contribute to the development of a retinal tear: Pathologic changes of the vitreous or increased vulnerability of the retinal tissues in cystoid degeneration (Fig. 121), in old age, in high myopia, aphakia or trauma.

Loss of vitreous, contracture of strands after trauma, hemorrhages and inflammations (proliferative retinopathy, exudative retinitis, periphlebitis) or subretinal hemorrhages, exudations or parasites as well as retinal and choroidal tumors may lead to *secondary* retinal detachment (page 164).

The pull on the retinal tissue causes the first *symptoms*, such as seeing dots, lightning streaks and other photoptic phenomena. Then suddenly a marked deterioration of vision occurs as a curtain, shadow or veil that covers the visual field. The visual field opposite the segment of detachment will first be lost. The visual disturbances are less pronounced in the morning after a night's rest or after any period of time in the horizontal position. The symptoms become more severe during the course of the day. The condition is painless. Ophthalmoscopically one first sees fine retinal folds (Fig. 122), later a bullous detachment.

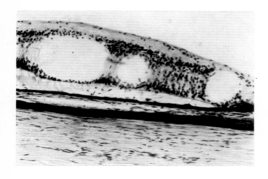

Fig. 121. Cystoid degeneration of the retinal periphery.

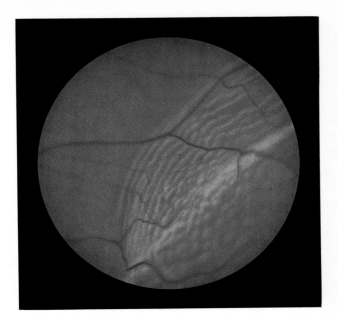

Fig. 122. Primary (serous) retinal detachment. Retinal folds are visible in the detached area. The blood vessels climb over the folds.

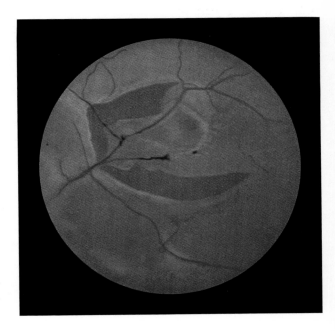

Fig. 123. Large horseshoe-shaped tear in the retinal periphery.

For treatment an exact localization of all retinal tears is mandatory. Only the closure of all holes (with diathermy, light coagulation, or cryotherapy, Fig. 124) will lead to a firm reattachment and scar formation (Fig. 125). Frequently it is necessary to complement these procedures by a scleral-buckling operation. In these operations a synthetic material or an autogenous substance is placed on the sclera in such a way that the sclera bulges toward the vitreous. This brings the choroid closer to the retina. The prognosis of a retinal detachment depends upon its early treatment and upon the number and location of the holes. Additional factors are the status of the retina and the vitreous.

Ophthalmoscopic Finding (Figs. 122–125)

Disc:	Normal color and sharply outlined.
Vessels:	Tortuous, conspicuously dark, elevated over the normal retinal level.
Retina:	Either flat detachment with the retina slightly wavy and transparent (Fig. 122); or the detachment is bullous, high and stiff. The detached retina appears greyish-green as the red of the choroid does not shine through.
	Tears in the retina appear bright red (Figs. 123, 124) with white margins; they are usually tongue- or horseshoe-shaped. The horseshoe is open toward the periphery and the operculum is lifted into the vitreous.
Choroid:	In myopic patients circumpapillary and central choroidal atrophy (Fig. 117).

Differential Diagnosis

Solid Detachment (Neoplasm) (page 164).
Subretinal Hemorrhage (Fig. 148). Subretinal Exudation.

The following examination methods may be used for differential diagnosis: Trans-scleral illumination (page 28), radioactive isotopes (^{32}P) which accumulate in neoplastic tissue, fluorescein angiography, and the echogram obtained on ultrasonographic examination. The latter is especially important to differentiate a serous from a solid detachment. It is a particularly valuable method since it can be used even when the media are completely opaque.

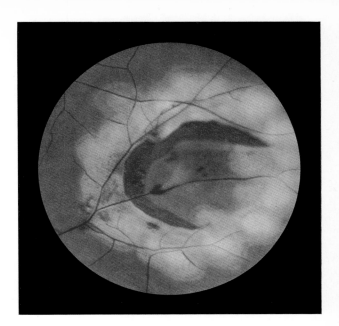

Fig. 124. Horseshoe-shaped tear surrounded by light co-agulation.

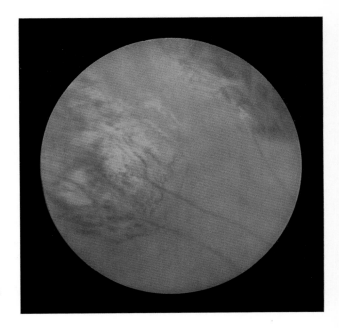

Fig. 125. Chorioretinitic scars after detachment operation.

10. Coats' Disease

General

In Coats' disease we find pre-, intra- and subretinal hemorrhages and transudations. This is followed by scar-tissue formation and secondary detachment. Histologically and histochemically one finds cholesterol and cholesterol-esters in the deposits lying in the deep retinal layers and beneath the retina. There are also foam cells and unsaturated fatty acids present.

The disease predominantly affects young males. Sometimes both eyes are affected. The etiology is undetermined.

Ophthalmoscopic Finding

Disc: Blurred margins because of edema.
Vessels: Obscured by the edema or tortuous, with constrictions and
            dilatations, elevated over the retinal level, neovascularization and
            multiple aneurysms.
Retina: Yellowish-grey with folds, irregular edematous areas, retinal and
            subretinal hemorrhages, glistening deposits (cholesterol crystals)
            and light degenerative areas.

Differential Diagnosis

Retinoblastoma (page 146).
Retinal angiomas (page 148)

11. Retrolental Fibroplasia

General

This is a disease of prematurely born infants with a birth weight of less than $4^1/_2$ pounds. If they remain in incubators with high oxygen concentration for a certain period of time, they will experience, upon exposure to normal oxygen tension, a short-lasting secondary oxygen deficiency of the not fully-developed retina. This oxygen deficiency has a certain toxic and stimulative effect upon the not fully-developed retinal vessels. There is first a constriction of these vessels and later a compensatory dilatation with proliferation of newly formed vessels, hemorrhages, and transudations into the vitreous. This may lead to connective tissue formation, shrinkage, membrane formation behind the lens and retinal detachment. A complicated cataract, secondary glaucoma or atrophy of the globe may lead to blindness.

Ophthalmoscopic Finding

(usually bilateral)

Early Stage: Attenuation of the arterioles, dilatation of the veins, retinal hemorrhages; later dilatation of all the vessels, opacification and detachment of the retinal periphery.

Around the Third Month: Proliferation of vessels into the vitreous, formation of connective tissue and scar tissue back of the lens.

Differential Diagnosis

Retinoblastoma (page 146).
Congenital malformations.
Pseudoglioma (page 147).

12. Neoplasms

a) Retinoblastoma

General

Retinoblastoma is a congenital neoplasm which consists of undifferentiated retinal elements. It is a disease of infancy and occurs in about a third of the cases bilaterally. Frequently the diagnosis is made only when the tumor fills a large

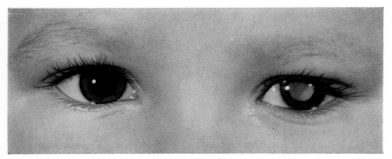

Fig. 126. Retinoblastoma appearing as an amaurotic cat's eye.

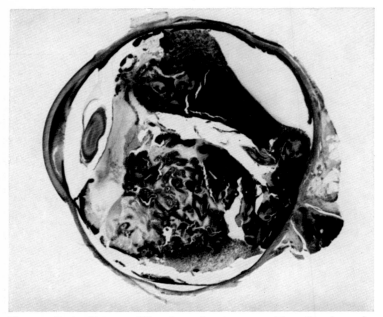

Fig. 127. Retinoblastoma filling the entire vitreous and invading the optic nerve.

part of the vitreous (Fig. 127) and causes a golden-yellow reflex in the pupillary area (amaurotic cat's eye) (Fig. 126). Later on the tumor will grow leading to secondary glaucoma and pain. The tumor grows relatively fast either along the optic nerve into the brain or through the coats of the eyeball into the orbit. It metastasizes to many other organs. Histologically one sees cords of large cells, often arranged around vessels, or the so-called rosettes.

Ophthalmoscopic Finding (Fig. 128)

Disc: Normal color and sharp outlines.
Retina: There is one or there are several greyish-white, sharply outlined nodules with irregular surface.

Differential Diagnosis

Pseudoglioma (These are congenital anomalies or sequelae of intraocular inflammation with scar tissue formation, as in metastatic ophthalmia).
Coats' Disease (page 144).
Retrolental Fibroplasia (page 145).

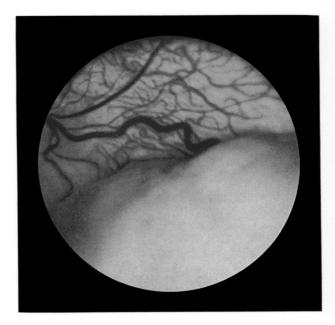

Fig. 128. Retinoblastoma. Grey-white tumor nodule growing into the vitreous.

b) Other Tumors

Tumor-like malformations can be found in the retina in some congenital, ectodermal dysplastic diseases, the so-called *phakomatoses* (VAN DER HOEVE). These retinal lesions occur together with pathologic changes in the brain and in other organs. They may be found in neurofibromatosis (von Recklinghausen disease) and Sturge-Weber disease.

Retinal angiomas or aneurysms together with arteriovenous anastomoses occur in *retinocerebral angiomatoses* (VON HIPPEL-LINDAU). Initially, markedly dilated and tortuous vessels (arteries and veins) are noted. At their peripheral termination is a dark-red, spheric nodule. Later on hemorrhages occur together with exudation and proliferation and finally a retinal detachment will ensue. In addition, angiomas are found in the cerebellum and in other organs.

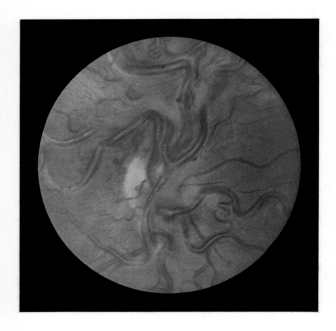

Fig. 129. Retinal angiomatosis: Conspicuous dilatation and tortuosity of the retinal vessels.

Multiple, small, mulberry-like tumors are found in the retina and especially close to the disc in tuberous sclerosis (BOURNEVILLE). This is a hereditary disease with a dominant gene (Fig. 130). In addition, there are pathologic changes of the skin and mucous membranes (sebaceous adenoma of Pringle). These are angiofibromas, small nodules covered by yellow-red telangiectasia occurring around the mouth and the nose. Parenchymatous organs (heart, kidneys) and the bones may be affected. Close to the cerebral ventricles or in the cerebral cortex are usually multiple tumors which frequently calcify. Even in childhood these lesions lead to epileptic seizures. There is frequently mental retardation, though some patients may be of normal intelligence.

Ophthalmoscopic Finding (Fig. 130)

Disc: Normal color and sharp outlines.
Vessels: Normal.
Retina: There is one large or several small, opaque, white nodules with mulberry-like surface.

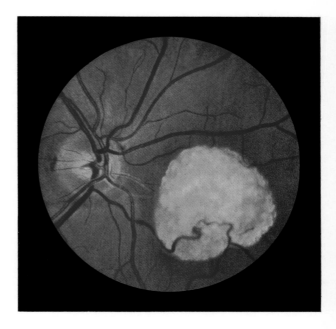

Fig. 130. Retinal tumor in tuberous sclerosis (Bourneville disease). White nodules with uneven surface are found close to the disc. The retinal vessels course over the nodule.

13. Injuries

General

Berlin's edema occurs after a *blunt injury* (page 130). It is usually transient and lasts only a few days. Ophthalmoscopically one sees a greyish-white opacification of the retinal tissues. The opaque area is of varying size and situated mainly at the posterior pole or in the periphery depending on the kind and effect of the force (Fig. 131). Usually the retina recovers completely and promptly. Occasionally a macular hole (page 131, Fig. 114) and rarely a retinal detachment (page 140) may follow.

Ophthalmoscopic Finding (Fig. 131)

Disc: Normal color and sharp outlines.
Vessels: (Transiently) attenuated.
Retina: Circumscribed, greyish-white edema in the area of the contre-coup.
            Occasionally small hemorrhages and fine folds.

Severe contusions, for instance bullet injuries to the orbit, may lead to extensive retinal and choroidal hemorrhages which after months are transformed into large pigmented scars and strands *(retinitis sclopetaria)* (Fig. 132).

Ophthalmoscopic Finding (Fig. 132)

Disc: Normal color. The disc may be pale if there is a simultaneous traumatic damage to the optic nerve.
Vessels: Unchanged.
Retina: In the acute stage there are numerous pre- and intraretinal hemorrhages. Later, there are large areas of brown-black pigmented scars.

Perforating injuries may lead to the introduction of a metallic foreign body into the eye. If such foreign bodies cannot be removed, they may lead to deposition of iron (siderosis) or copper (chalcosis) and to blindness.

A retina may suffer from distant injuries such as *compression of the thorax*. This may lead to retinal hemorrhages and opacities along the veins *(Purtscher's disease)*. These are probably due to fat emboli or stasis in the vessels. They disappear within a few weeks.

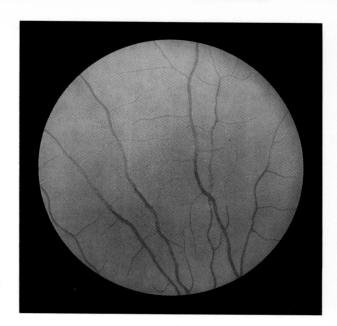

Fig. 131. Berlin's edema: In the upper segment after blunt injury to the globe by a fist.

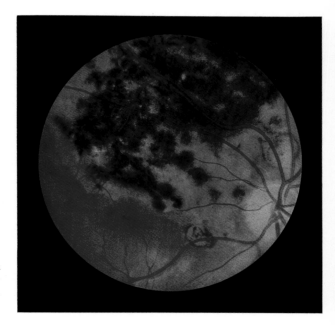

Fig. 132. Retinitis sclopetaria after contusion of the globe by a football; extensive, pigmented scars.

VIII. Diseases of the Choroid

1. Inflammatory Diseases

General

An inflammation of the choroid is often due to a systemic disease which spreads via the blood stream (tuberculosis, rheumatism, syphilis, bacterial infections). Such an inflammation (choroiditis) is painless. It has a chronic course with many exacerbations and remissions. One, therefore, frequently finds old scar tissue in addition to fresh infiltrates. According to the number of inflammatory foci we distinguish *isolated* (Figs. 133–136, 139), *disseminated* (irregularly distributed foci, Fig. 137) and *diffuse* choroiditis (when large areas are involved, Fig. 138). According to the localization of the infiltrate we distinguish between a central and a peripheral chorioretinitis. In the course of time both eyes may become involved. Choroiditis may be accompanied by an anterior uveitis (iritis, iridocyclitis) with opacities in the aqueous and vitreous. Depending upon the number and localization of inflammatory foci the retinal function may be disturbed. Peripheral changes may cause hemeralopia and constriction of the visual field. Foci at the posterior pole will produce a decrease in visual acuity. The disease is often recognized only when a focus involves the macular area (page 129).

In acute miliary tuberculosis one frequently sees numerous small greyish-white infiltrates with blurred outlines disseminated over the entire eyeground.

The ophthalmoscopic picture of a choroiditis – independent from its etiology – usually consists of *large* areas of involvement and *coarse* pigmentation (this is in contrast to the small areas involved in *retinopathy,* page 89).

It is of great importance to decide whether we are dealing with a fresh infiltrate or an old, healed scar.

Fresh infiltrates are grey to green with fluffy borders and are slightly elevated.

Old scars are sharply outlined and yellow-white, since the choroid is atrophic and the white sclera shines through.

The retina is primarily not involved and hemorrhages are usually absent.

The inflammation causes a secondary proliferation of the retinal pigment epithelium and the chorioretinic scar is, therefore, often surrounded by coarse pigmentation. These changes require a certain period of time and a *fresh focus* of choroiditis is *never pigmented.*

The pigmentation is especially coarse in *syphilitic chorioretinitis.* At the same time we may find here edematous changes at the disc and in the retina.

a) Acute Choroiditis

> Isolated (central, peripheral).
> Disseminated.
> Diffuse.

Ophthalmoscopic Finding (Figs. 133–135)

Disc: Sharp margins; only when the choroiditis is juxtapapillary may the margins be blurred.

Choroidal Infiltrate:

Size: Relatively large plaques or dots.

Color: Dirty yellow to grey-green.

Form: Varies.

Margins: Fluffy.

Vessels: Primarily not affected; the retinal vessels may be seen elevated because of the choroidal infiltrate.

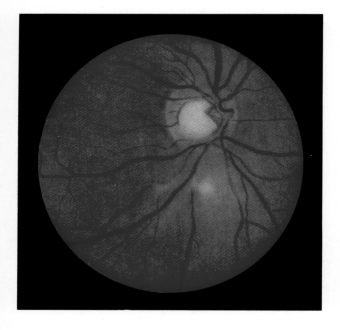

Fig. 133. Acute, isolated choroiditis. Circumscribed, grey, edematous area at the inferior temporal artery close to the disc; large physiologic excavation.

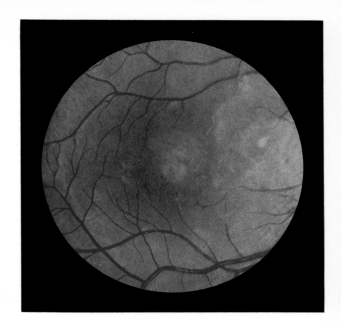

Fig. 134. Acute, circumscribed, central choroiditis. Dirty-grey edema in the macula.

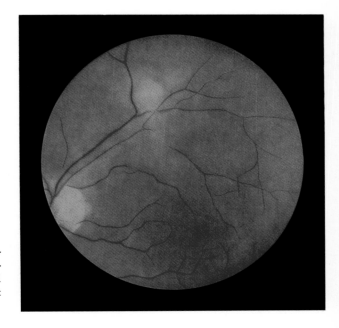

Fig. 135. Subacute circumscribed, choroiditis. The inflammatory area is already well circumscribed, but not yet pigmented.

b) Old Choroiditis

Ophthalmoscopic Finding (Figs. 136–138)

Disc: Normal; partial pallor only with juxtapapillary choroiditis.
Choroidal Focus:
Size: Large area involved.
Color: Yellow-white, pigmentation at the margin or centrally.
Form: Varies.
Margins: Sharp.
Vessels: Not affected.

Differential Diagnosis

Choroidal Coloboma (page 49).
Macular Degeneration (page 128).
Myopic Choroidal Degenerations (page 134).
Contusion and Rupture of the Choroid (page 168).

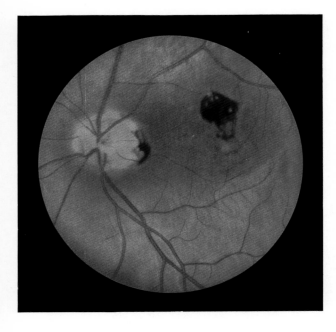

Fig. 136. Old central, isolated choroiditis. Pigmented scar in and above the macula.

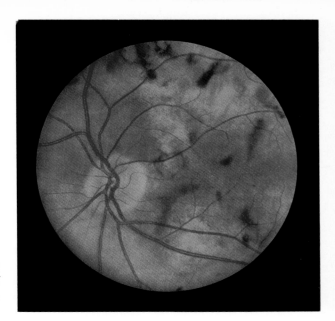

Fig. 137. Old disseminated choroiditis. Numerous areas of choroidal atrophy and scars, partly pigmented.

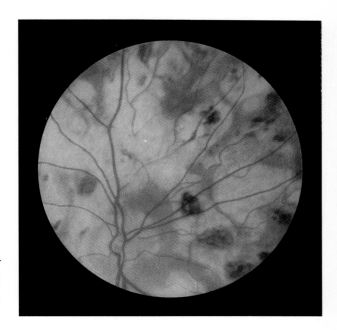

Fig. 138. Old diffuse choroiditis. The inflammatory areas are sharply outlined and partly pigmented. The light sclera shines through.

c) Chorioretinitis

Inflammatory conditions of choroid and retina are called chorioretinitis.

α) Juxtapapillary Chorioretinitis (Jensen)

General

In this condition we have next to the optic nervehead an inflammatory focus in the choroid. Because of severe involvement of the retina a sector-shaped visual field defect will be present. This visual defect begins at the blind spot and reaches the periphery in an arcuate form.

Ophthalmoscopic Finding (Fig. 139)

Disc: Edematous, partly blurred margins.

Retina and Choroid: Circumscribed retinal edema, beneath it greyish-white fluffy choroidal focus (usually next to the disc).

In the *end-stage* one finds a sharply outlined, coarsely pigmented scar with choroidal atrophy and sclera shining through it.

β) Toxoplasmosis

General

In patients with typical *congenital* toxoplasmosis we find an internal hydrocephalus, cerebral calcifications, and often bilateral scars in the macular area. The macular lesions resemble a pseudocoloboma. They are the scars of an old, central chorioretinitis. They cause a marked decrease in visual acuity. Infants with nystagmus or suspected poor vision should be examined as early as possible with the ophthalmoscope. Only rarely are similar changes found in the periphery of the fundus. In exacerbations "retinal satellites" may appear at the margin of the congenital scar.

The disease is caused by the intra-uterine infection with the parasite Toxoplasma gondii. The verification of the diagnosis can only be made with immunologic tests measuring the presence of antibodies in blood and aqueous (methylene blue) test.

Ophthalmoscopic Finding (Fig. 140)

Disc: Normal color and sharply outlined.

Vessels: Frequently irregular.

Retina and Choroid: Initially circumscribed edema in the macular area; later pigmented atrophic scar.

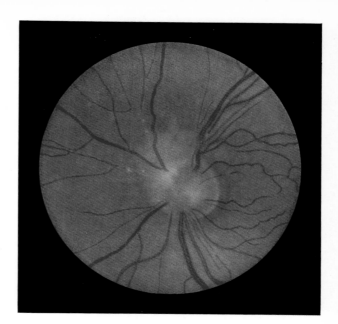

Fig. 139. Juxtapapillary chorio-retinitis. The upper margin of the disc is blurred. A grey, recent inflammatory focus lies immediately adjacent to the disc.

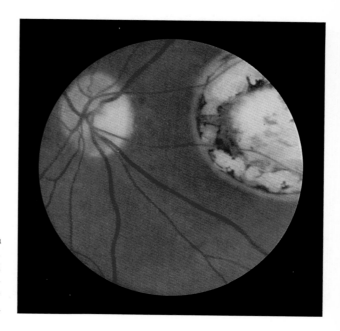

Fig. 140. Central choroiditis in congenital toxoplasmosis. Large sharply demarcated and pigmented area of chorio-retinal atrophy at the posterior pole in the area of the macula.

Differential Diagnosis

Choroidal Coloboma (page 51).

Central Chorioretinitis of another cause (page 153).

In *acquired* toxoplasmosis, close to the disc we find at first yellow-brown, later grey-brown isolated retinal foci with a slight elevation and marginal hemorrhages. These lesions are rarer and less pathognomonic than the ones found in congenital toxoplasmosis.

γ) Syphilitic Chorioretinitis

General

Because of a syphilitic vasculitis the fundus will show bilateral pigmentations and depigmentations (salt and pepper fundus). These changes occur in *congenital* syphilis mostly in the periphery.

In the *acquired* forms the pigmentation is coarser than in the congenital type.

At the same time there frequently are vitreous opacities, vascular changes (endarteritis), and optic atrophy present.

Ophthalmoscopic Finding

Disc: Normal color or pale, sharply outlined.

Retina: Irregularly distributed small light retinitic foci with fine pigmentary disturbances.

Choroid: Atrophic.

δ) Central Serous Retinopathy

General

In this condition we find a circumscribed edema in the area of the posterior pole. The cause is an inflammatory process in the choriocapillaries producing a swelling of the overlying retina. Characteristic is a leakage of fluid through a break in the pigment epithelium. This leak is well visible on fluorescein angiography. Corresponding to the damage in the macular area there will be loss of central visual acuity, a positive central scotoma, micropsia, metamorphopsia, chromatopsia, and a transient hyperopia as the retinal edema shortens the optical axis (page 21). Most often affected are males from twenty-five to fifty years old. This disease has a tendency to recur. The subretinal fluid may sink downward and become absorbed. With this all symptoms disappear. Occasionally the leak has to be sealed with light coagulation.

Ophthalmoscopic Finding

Disc: Normal color, sharply outlined.

Retina and Choroid: Circumscribed edema in the macular area surrounded by light reflexes. Slight elevation; later light dots (precipitates on the retina), and slight pigmentations.

2. Degenerative Diseases

Degenerative processes of the choroid occur with mechanical stretching (page 61), chronic disturbances of the blood supply, or as a hereditary disease.

a) Choroidal Sclerosis

General

Advanced arteriosclerosis, which often also affects the retinal vessels, will lead to corresponding changes of the choroidal vessels (see "senile macular degeneration," page 132).

Ophthalmoscopic Finding (Fig. 141)

Disc: Normal.
Vessels: Arteriosclerosis (page 104).
Retina: Disappearance of pigment epithelium.
Choroid: The choroidal vessels are visible especially close to the disc or in the macular area. They appear like bright red ribbons, or like a white-yellow net because of multiple occlusions. The brownish intervascular spaces are well visible with the white sclera shining through; pigmentary disturbances.

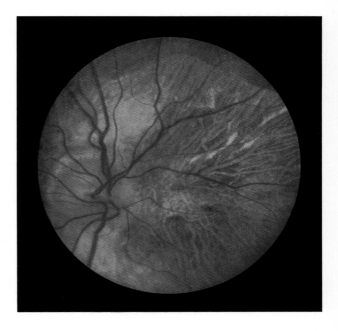

Fig. 141. Choroidal sclerosis: Choroidal vessels are well visible, partly occluded.

b) Drusen of Bruch's Membrane

These appear as small, light atrophic areas, often at the posterior pole. They correspond to excrescences of Bruch's membrane and are deposits of hyaline or calcium (Fig. 142). These structures may cause pressure atrophy of the pigment epithelium, and if they are large enough and situated in the fovea, even disturbances of visual function.

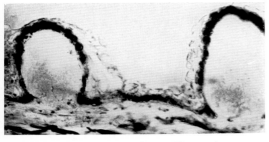

Fig.142. Drusen of Bruch's membrane (photomicrograph).

Ophthalmoscopic Finding (Fig. 143)

Disc: Normal color and sharply outlined.

Retina and Choroid: Usually on the temporal side are yellowish-white, sometimes glistening, small foci. They are often arranged in groups. They have a sharp outline.

Differential Diagnosis

Degenerative Foci in Arteriosclerosis of Hypertonic Fundus (pages 102, 108). Macular Diseases (page 128).

c) Choroideremia

Choroideremia is a progressive choroidal atrophy which belongs to the tapeto-retinal degenerations (page 135). It begins in the periphery and leads to hemeralopia and constriction of the visual field. In the early stages the macula and the area around the disc are spared. Later, the choroid becomes atrophic in these areas also. The clinical picture may resemble that of the gyrate atrophy of choroid and retina. It is a sex-linked recessive hereditary disease affecting only males. Blindness is the usual end-result.

Ophthalmoscopic Finding (Fig. 144)

Disc: Normal.

Retina: Normal.

Choroid: Has largely disappeared. The fundus shows no details and appears light as the sclera shines through. A few bone-corpuscle-like pigmentations are distributed irregularly.

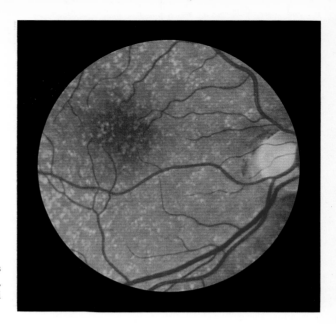

Fig. 143. Drusen of Bruch's membrane. Numerous small, light, somewhat elevated foci at the posterior pole.

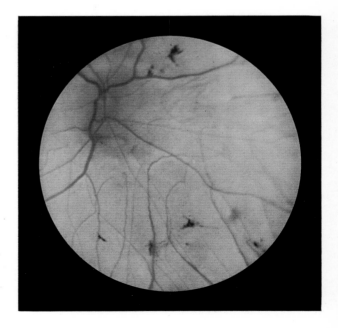

Fig. 144. Choroideremia. Extreme atrophy of the choroid. The sclera shines through. A few bone-corpuscle-like pigmentations are visible.

3. Neoplasms

a) Benign Neoplasms

The only benign neoplasms of the choroid are nevi (page 59) and hemangiomas. The latter are rare. They are usually situated close to the disc and may be accompanied by a hemangioma of the face (nevus flammeus). They may cause a retinal detachment and secondary glaucoma. Their differential diagnosis from a melanoma may be difficult (page 166).

b) Malignant Neoplasms

α) Melanoma

General

The most frequent primary tumor of the uveal tract is the melanoma. It occurs about ten times more often in the choroid than in the iris or the ciliary body.

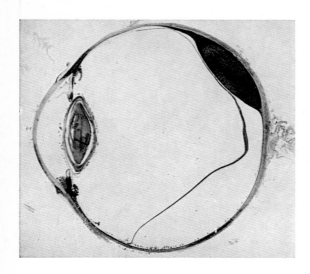

Fig. 145. Melanoma of the choroid.

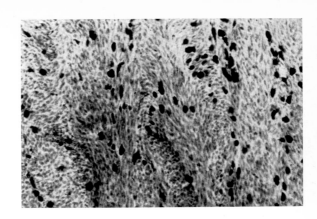

Fig. 146. Choroidal melanoma (photomicrograph).

It is a disease of adulthood and is practically always *unilateral*. The symptoms depend upon the size and location of the tumor. If the tumor lies in the periphery of the choroid, it will cause symptoms only when it has reached a considerable size. In melanomas of the *iris* we often find changes of the pupil and disturbances of pupillary reactions. In melanomas of the *ciliary body* the lens may be subluxated and there may be a marked difference between the intraocular pressure of the healthy and the affected eye. *Choroidal* melanomas will lead to a retinal detachment and corresponding visual disturbances and defects of the visual field. The tumor may grow flat toward the sides (Fig. 145) or more often, like a mushroom through a break in Bruch's membrane into the subretinal space. It may extend along vessels and nerves into and through the sclera to the orbit. The tumor metastasizes via the blood stream into other organs (liver, lungs and bones). According to the cell type we distinguish histologically spindle and epithelioid cell melanomas. The degree of pigmentation may vary from dark black to absent pigmentation (Fig. 146). The prognosis varies according to size, extension, cell type, and degree of pigmentation.

The final diagnosis may not be possible during the early stages on the basis of the ophthalmoscopic picture alone. Supplementary examination methods may be necessary to make an early diagnosis, such as scleral transillumination (page 28), fluorescein angiography, the accumulation of radioactive substance (^{32}P) or the echogram with ultrasound.

Ophthalmoscopic Finding (Fig. 147)

Disc: Normal color and sharply outlined.
Vessels: Tortuous, elevated over the lesion.
Retina: Circumscribed detachment, appears brownish-grey, pigment may
                 appear on the surface and at the margin of the detachment.

Differential Diagnosis

Choroidal Nevus (page 59): Here the patient has to be observed in order to see changes in the lesion, fundus photography may be necessary.

Subretinal Hemorrhage (Fig. 148).

Serous Retinal Detachment (page 140), cyst or hemangioma of the choroid, choroidal detachment.

β) Metastatic Tumors

General

Metastatic tumors of the choroid are due to the hematogenous dissemination of a carcinoma. The primary tumor is often a breast carcinoma. The metastatic tumor may also be secondary to a tumor of the lungs or the gastrointestinal tract. Many other carcinomas may on occasion metastasize into the highly vascularized choroid (for instance kidney, adrenals, prostate, thyroid, etc.). The symptoms of a metastatic choroidal tumor are not different from those of a primary melanoma. Secondary tumors frequently grow much faster than a melanoma. In addition, they have a tendency to become bilateral. The prognosis is extremely poor. Radiotherapy or systemic treatment is indicated (chemotherapy, hormonal therapy).

The histologic picture resembles that of the primary tumor.

Ophthalmoscopic Finding (Fig. 48)

Disc: Normal color and sharply outlined.
Vessels: Unchanged.
Retina and Choroid: Greyish-yellow, slightly elevated lesions are present in the
                 fundus. There may be radial folds next to them.

Differential Diagnosis

Choroidal melanoma (page 164), acute choroiditis (page 153).

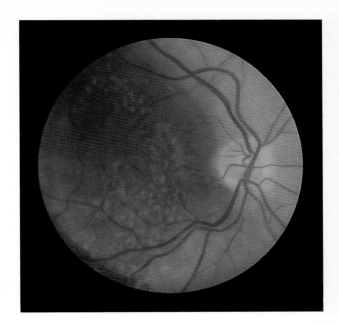

Fig. 147. Choroidal melanoma reaching the temporal disc margin.

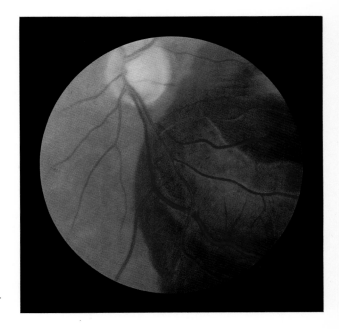

Fig. 148. Subretinal hemorrhage.

4. Injuries (Choroidal Rupture)

General

In instances of severe blunt traumas to the eyeball, the choroid may show hemorrhages (Fig. 149) or tears. These appear either in the area where the force was applied or, as a "contre-coup" in a typical arcuate form at the posterior pole close to the disc. If the macula is involved (traumatic macular affection, page 150), a permanent, severe decrease in visual acuity will result. Sometimes we find several such ruptures next to each other.

Ophthalmoscopic Finding (Fig. 150)

Disc: Normal color and sharply outlined (if there is no traumatic damage to the optic nerve at the same time).

Vessels: Unchanged.

Retina and Choroid: Concentrically to the disc we find sickle-like cracks through which the white sclera is visible. In the beginning there are hemorrhages and retinal edema, later on pigmentation.

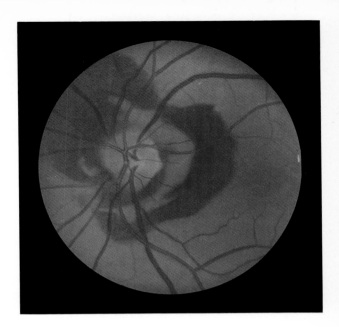

Fig. 149. Extensive peripapillary hemorrhages after contusion. The eye was hit with a fist.

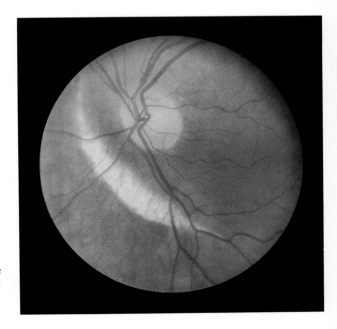

Fig. 150. Choroidal rupture nasally and below the disc. The white sclera shines through here.

Index